the 5 kinds of intimacy

HOW TO KEEP YOUR LOVE ALIVE

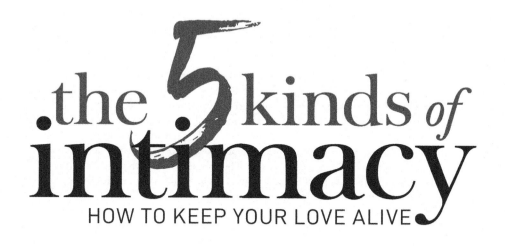

the 5 kinds of intimacy

HOW TO KEEP YOUR LOVE ALIVE

Beth Darling

Published by Darling Enterprises, LLC

Publishing Consultant:
Redwood Publishing, LLC
Orange County, California
www.redwooddigitalpublishing.com

Printed in the United States of America

ISBN: 978-1-956470-77-2 (hardcover)
ISBN: 978-1-956470-78-9 (paperback)
ISBN: 978-1-956470-79-6 (e-book)

Library of Congress Control Number: 2023901548

Cover Design by Michelle Manley of Graphique Designs, LLC
Front Cover Photo and Author Photo by Kelley Sweet Photography
Interior Design by Jose Pepito

Disclaimer: Please note that throughout the book the stories are based on truth, but names and identifying details have been changed, stories merged or compressed, and dialogue recreated. Any likeness is coincidental.

To my Aunt Cindy, who has always given me safe harbor despite the mess I create in her immaculate home. I'm forever impressed and grateful that she allowed our relationship to become infinitely more intimate and meaningful in the toughest of times.

CONTENTS

PART ONE
What You Need to Know About Intimacy

PART TWO
A Practical Playbook: Easy Intimacy Practices for Everyone

"If fear is the great enemy of intimacy, love is its true friend."

—Henri Nouwen

Love, Language, and Intimacy

It was obvious to all that George and Liz loved each other very much. They were kind, supportive, and warm with each other; no one could doubt they enjoyed being together. Most importantly, they both described their twenty-eight-year marriage as happy, which isn't all that common these days. Given this, you might be surprised to learn that they both felt something was lacking. When prompted, they admitted that the sparks had been gone for a while; they each had a feeling that while things certainly weren't bad, they weren't as close as they'd like to be. So, being the proactive, ambitious people they are (in love as well as in life), they decided to make some changes.

Toward that goal, they decided to read *The 5 Love Languages*®, Gary Chapman's bestselling book that's been a fan favorite—and recommended by therapists everywhere—for the past thirty years.[1] When they finished it, George and Liz committed themselves to ninety days of sharing love with their partner in the way their partner wanted to receive it. Since Liz liked words of affirmation, George gave her sincere compliments every day. He would tell her how attractive she was and

---

[1] Chapman pioneered the concept that there are five "languages," or ways, in which romantic partners give and receive love: words of affirmation, quality time, gifts, acts of service, and physical touch.

how much he enjoyed her cooking. Whenever he left the house to play a few rounds of golf, he would make sure to tell her how much he appreciated her taking care of the kids so he could spend time with his friends.

In return, Liz provided George with acts of service every day. She cooked him delicious meals, picked up his dry cleaning, and kept his favorite snacks stocked in the pantry—where their kids couldn't find them. Their two love languages flowed naturally between them; it was easy for George to verbally acknowledge (words of affirmation) Liz's thoughtful acts (acts of service).

But at the end of the ninety days, even though Liz and George agreed it had been a pleasant experience, they didn't feel anything significant had really changed or improved between them. They had been a bit nicer and more attentive to each other for three months, but they weren't any more passionate or excited to be together. They didn't feel any more "in love."

They wondered if this meant they were not meant to be together after all.

I was so glad George and Liz came to me after this experiment rather than throwing in the towel on what was clearly a loving relationship. It was obvious to me that they had some great tools (love languages), but they weren't using them effectively enough. They weren't yet using those tools to create what their relationship truly needed: intimacy.

For the past ninety days, they'd been using love languages to express their love for each other, which was great! But they didn't realize that as wonderful as love is, on its own, it lacks the substance—the *intimacy*—needed to make a relationship truly fulfilling.

I wish you could have seen the shock on their faces when the truth became obvious: they'd been loving each other throughout their entire marriage but were still "hungry" because they hadn't been focusing on intimacy!

Don't get me wrong; *The 5 Love Languages* is a fabulous resource. It has given millions of couples insight into how they enjoy giving and receiving love. Chapman gave the world a powerful tool kit. It's no wonder we all got so excited; we never stopped to question what to build with all the love we finally knew how to express!

It's as if we got new woodworking tools. Can you imagine spending years sawing wood into pieces, which you'd then hammer full of nails, only to throw them into a pile in the corner? Sure, that may be a fun activity when you're learning to use a new tool, but it doesn't take long before aimlessly hammering away becomes pretty boring. If, on the other hand, you focus on using your skills to create something substantive, like a bench to place under your favorite shade tree, you'll probably experience a burst of pride every time someone uses it. In turn, that feeling of success will likely motivate you to build something else.

What it boils down to is this: Love is an emotion. Love languages are tools we can use to express or receive that emotion, but that's not the end of the story. I see lots of loving marriages where each spouse is fluent in the other's love language, but far too many of these relationships are still suffering from a lack of intimacy. How do I know this? Think of all the married couples who live like roommates and/or operate like collegial business partners.

> Love languages are great tools we can use to create, build, and affirm intimacy. When both partners are receptive, a perpetual intimacy cycle results, which keeps their love alive.

In happy, lasting romantic relationships, love languages are used to create mutually fulfilling intimacy between loving partners. This not only sustains their existing love; it also spurs more intimacy, which, in turn, grows even more love.

In other words, love languages are great tools we can use to create, build, and affirm intimacy. When both partners are receptive, a perpetual intimacy cycle results, which keeps their love alive.

Now, I get it; talk is cheap. It's easy to say, "Yay, let's build intimacy!" just like it's easy to say, "Let's build a table." But when push comes to shove, at least we all know what a table is. While we may not know the exact steps involved in building one, we know what a table looks like and what it does: A table has legs that support a surface upon which we can place other items. When it comes to intimacy, on the other hand, we're pretty much clueless. We're not sure what it looks like, what it's made of, or what its purpose is. We've never learned a clear-cut, concise, workable definition of intimacy. Nor have we ever had a specific understanding of the role intimacy plays in our relationships. No wonder we've been frustrated! No wonder so many people have "settled."

Personally, I found the circular, illogical uses of the term *intimacy* so unhelpful that I had to unravel it before I drove myself nuts! I have no sense of direction but going in circles isn't fun for anyone. Thankfully, I have a mind skilled in getting to the root of an issue and loves logic problems, so the geeky part of me enjoyed the challenge. I figured understanding intimacy had to be easier than taking two different state bar exams, and I was right! My logical lawyer brain kicked into action as I searched desperately for a good working model of intimacy, and when I didn't find it, I created it.

My 5 Kinds of Intimacy are simple, easy to understand, fun to implement, and allow for insightful analysis. (The latter is key because it means we can identify what's working and what needs improvement.)

This book is devoted to clarifying, exploring, and celebrating these intimacies as the fundamental building blocks of a happy, lasting relationship. The ongoing creation and sharing of these intimacies are critical to any healthy, happy relationship.

Let's go back to George and Liz. When George was giving Liz words of affirmation, he was giving voice to his appreciation of her, which is lovely. But if he had focused on using his words of affirmation to create *intimacy*, they would have been significantly more impactful.

It's the difference between saying "thank you" while standing in the doorway when your neighbor brings you cookies and inviting them into your home for a cup of coffee.

Which of these do you think is better: A or B?

A. "It was so nice of you to pick up my dry cleaning today! You rock."

B. "When I was driving to work this morning, I felt so overwhelmed. I couldn't imagine how I'd get everything done before my big meeting. When I realized I could ask for your help, even though you had a busy day too, it made me feel truly loved. I've been killing it at work ever since. Now, instead of being worried about the meeting, I just can't wait to get home so I can hug you. You make my life better in big and little ways. Thank you, Lizzie! I love you always."

How do you think Liz is going to respond to A? To B?

Option A is fine—but utterly unremarkable. It's not going to push George and Liz apart, but it's also not likely to pull them together . . . unless they're so starved for any recognition or connection that they'll settle for crumbs.

(By the way, that was me for twenty-three years, so I'm not judging here! I'm just trying to help you avoid the same pain.)

In Option B, George is creating a big healthy dose of emotional intimacy by doing the following:

1) Being vulnerable:
   a) Exposing his feelings
   b) Needing and wanting her help

2) Recognizing that she has important things that matter to her, yet she prioritized him when he needed her, sacrificing some items on her own to-do list in order to do so

3) Letting her know her contribution enabled him to do better, which was meaningful

4) Affirming that being with her is important to his overall happiness

See the difference?

After working with thousands of couples, I have found that these 5 intimacies create love, passion, commitment, empathy, and compassion. Our willingness to be intimate expands our feelings of love as we joyfully lean into the value it adds to our lives. Shared intimacy with a loved one allows us to foster more trust, strengthen our connection, and grow closer.

This may *sound* grandiose, but it doesn't have to be. As Dr. John Gottman says, "Trust is built in the smallest of moments."[2] Intimacy is built there too.

In the past, our lack of clarity around intimacy meant we didn't know what the small pieces of intimacy were or how they worked together to create something greater. Today, it's easy to understand that the 5 intimacies are to a marriage like the food groups are to a body: Each one is

> These 5 intimacies create love, passion, commitment, empathy, and compassion. Our willingness to be intimate expands our feelings of love as we joyfully lean into the value it adds to our lives. Shared intimacy with a loved one allows us to foster more trust, strengthen our connection, and grow closer.

---

[2] Dr. John Gottman is world-renowned for his work on marital stability and divorce prediction. He's the author of over two hundred published academic articles and the author/coauthor of more than forty books, including the *New York Times* bestseller *The Seven Principles for Making Marriage Work.*

necessary. If a relationship is deprived of any one intimacy, it is more likely to wither away.

I don't want your love to wither. I want it to thrive so that it sustains and fulfills you throughout your life. In this book, I'll teach you how to create a healthy diet that includes each kind of intimacy. You'll learn what part each plays in a healthy partnership so you'll understand the benefits, as well as notice the signs of a deficit. Next, I'll give you a straightforward worksheet to assess what's working—or not working—in your relationship. Lastly, you'll find a bunch of simple, fun practices to easily create more intimacy. The best part is these aren't "one and done" practices; you'll enjoy using them for years to come.

By the time you finish reading this book, you should be not only fluent in the languages of love but also skilled in using them to create intimacy that will keep your love alive.

INTRODUCTION

You're Made for Love

My name is Beth Darling—a.k.a. Beth Liebling[3]—and, to the endless mortification of my five children, I like to talk about sexy fun.

I don't mean I like to talk about it every once in a while or subtly. No, I mean I like to talk about sexy fun at full volume, unashamed, whenever and wherever the need or urge arises—whether it's at the dinner table, a wedding reception, or even church or temple. (Today, it was in the American Express Centurion Lounge at the Denver International Airport.)

I guess I'm a bit of a rebel. I like tackling issues that others shy away from, especially when those issues include the possibility of great pleasure!

To me, sexy stuff is the huge, hidden base of the relationship iceberg that people don't like to talk about. The problem is if an iceberg can sink the *Titanic*, imagine the damage it can do to an unsuspecting couple. I have a bit more experience with this than I'd like, frankly. Which probably explains why I talk about sexy stuff with such glee;

---

[3] My birth name is Beth Liebling, but it's hard to spell. Since Liebling means *darling* in German, I simplify things by using Beth Darling. :-)

once I realized there was the possibility of endless, guilt-free, healthy, happy PLEASURE waiting for us below the surface, how could I resist?

Plus, I've found that it's actually quite fun to be comfortable with stuff that makes other people nervous. I adore helping others through the awkwardness by laughing *with* them, never *at* them. After all, if we want healthy, happy, lasting relationships, we've gotta deal with sex, so we might as well enjoy it!

That being said, let's not ignore the rest of the iceberg. That's why you're reading this book, right? You don't want just a piece of a good relationship; you want it all! You want the secret recipe that will keep your love alive.

Forgive me for chuckling, but the irony is I'm a terrible cook. Don't worry, though; I'm really good at teaching people how to create passionate love! Maybe you've read my first book, *Love and Laughter: Sexy (Meaningful) Fun for Everyone.* Maybe you've heard me talk about intimacy on TV, podcasts, TikTok, or the radio. Maybe you've attended one of my many workshops on love, sex, and relationships. Or maybe we met at my beloved, oh-so-sexy Darling Way Boutique in Houston, Texas.[4] Or maybe you'd never heard of me until you discovered this book.

> You don't want just a piece of a good relationship; you want it all! You want the secret recipe that will keep your love alive.

However you got here, I'm thrilled. I'm honored by your trust. I give you my word that no matter how lighthearted my approach is, I take loving relationships seriously. Please remember this as we delve into some juicy conversations that may feel new, unusual, or even a little scary to you. That's exactly why you're here. That's why these topics are included in this book; if they're left unexamined, you're likely to crash into them with painful consequences. It's better that we have these

---

[4] I sold the shop in 2021 so that I could talk more about love, intimacy, and sexy stuff, as opposed to spending all my time in retail management.

conversations together so you'll be more equipped to handle whatever roadblocks you'll face down the road. I hope that instead of resisting the parts of this book that stir up difficult emotions for you, you'll realize that those are the places where you should throw on your invisible cloak of courage and dive right in. Those are the sections that will most likely be the most impactful for you. They'll probably feel the most emotionally intimate, which is good, even if it's difficult.

Intimacy is, after all, the point of this book.

If lasting love, a happy marriage, and/or family values matter to you, intimacy should matter. (By the way, when I use the term *family values*, I mean celebrating the benefits of a happy, loving family, whether formed by blood or choice, without limitation.) Heck, even if you just want to be a happy hermit, self-intimacy is going to be key!

But while intimacy is my focus in this book, I never lose sight of why it's so important. It's because of love.

That's why I'm here. Love is my jam! I am a hopeful, shameless romantic who believes in lasting, fulfilling, passionately exciting love. I believe all of us deserve to experience it. I believe all of us *can* experience it, even though no one's ever taught us how to do so! Love is a magical recipe; each individual chef is responsible for creating their own unique version. They might start with the same basic ingredients, but there are endless possibilities. Each must experiment to create exactly what they want.

It's no wonder I became very interested in that recipe. Once I started to look, really *look* at the most vibrant, loving romantic relationships I could find—among my clients, my friends, even myself—to understand

> If lasting love, a happy marriage, and/or family values matter to you, intimacy should matter. (By the way, when I use the term *family values*, I mean celebrating the benefits of a happy, loving family whether formed by blood or choice, without limitation.)

what they had that others lacked, I kept coming back to one word: intimacy.

I'd spent years teaching the pleasure of sexy fun in my workshops, helping thousands of couples improve their sex lives by improving their communication skills while strengthening their emotional connection, but there were still pieces missing from their relationships. Sure, sexual intimacy was an obvious place to start; that's why so many people came to see me. But there was more to the story. And I love a good story!

So I dug deeper. It didn't take me long to realize there wasn't just one kind of intimacy; it was more complex. I almost surprised myself when it occurred to me that not only could we experience it with our partners, but we could also experience it with total strangers! Even involuntarily!

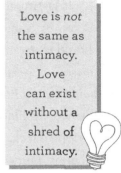

Love is *not* the same as intimacy. Love can exist without a shred of intimacy.

At some point early on, the following idea became apparent to me: Love is *not* the same as intimacy. But I didn't find that too shocking.

Wanna know what completely took me by surprise?

Love can exist without a shred of intimacy.

That blew my mind.

It changed everything for me.

As I began to tease apart the kinds of intimacy, a new theory knit itself together in my brain. From there, I started to see the ways in which different kinds of intimacy are essential—why the most fulfilling relationships need all of them to thrive.

Suddenly, every client I worked with, every couple I coached, even the relationships I saw in my personal life—not to mention my own life—looked different. I had a new framework through which to under-stand the dynamics. The strengths and the weaknesses in each relation-ship became almost glaringly obvious. Through this lens I could see *how* some loves lasted and *why* other loves died on the vine. I watched some couples grow closer with intimacy while others worked hard to avoid it. I watched some people's love get stronger while others deteriorated over time. I even came to understand why some loving relationships didn't last.[5]

I finally had all the pieces of the puzzle. I had unlocked the secret to deep, lasting, passionate relationships. The key is intimacy—specifically, five kinds of it:

1. Physical Intimacy

Physical intimacy can include touching—a hug, a hand on the small of the back, a caress on the cheek. But it is also created when someone, even a stranger, invades your personal space via their proximity. For example, you experience physical intimacy when squeezed into a crowded elevator or train. We'll cozy up to this kind of intimacy, taking a closer look at how to cultivate awareness around physical intimacy in our love relationships by tuning in—and turning on.

2. Emotional Intimacy

When we reveal our—or witness someone else's—emotional vulnerability, their deepest feelings, fears, hopes, dreams, or dread, **emotional intimacy** is created. In these moments, one's inner self is seen or exposed, regardless of whether or not it's acknowledged. This can occur via conversation, tears, emotional outbursts, or other vulnerable expressions of self—even if we aren't seeking intimacy! As we move forward, we'll dig into all the feelings this brings up before addressing ways to *choose* to be emotionally intimate as a path to deeper connection.

---

[5] By the way, whether or not you prefer monogamy is irrelevant in my mind. Gay, straight, polyamorous—I love and support them all! I just want whatever relationship(s) you choose to be wholly fulfilling and satisfying, with plenty of love and intimacy.

3. Sexual Intimacy

Believe it or not, **sexual intimacy** isn't just about sex. Yes, there is sexual intimacy when people engage in sexual acts with others. But we also have sexual intimacy with our gynecologist or proctologist, even our platonic friends! We'll romp into all this, as well as *intentional* sexy fun, snuggling up to some surprising truths about how sexual intimacy plays out in relationships and when it's cheating or not. We'll discuss why it doesn't always require physical intimacy; participating in phone sex, cybersex, and conversations *about* sex, even hearing other people have sex, are sexually intimate acts as well.

4. Romantic Intimacy

Romantic intimacy is the energy, ambiance, excitement, or surprise that elevates an experience from ordinary to extraordinary. It's a picnic under the Eiffel Tower versus a picnic in your backyard. It may or may not occur in conjunction with sexual intimacy. We'll discover the ways our cultural idea of "romance"—spending money on luxury items such as flowers, jewelry, etc.—is different from romantic intimacy. We'll discover the ingredients needed to create actual romance, not just the pretense of romance.

5. Spiritual Intimacy

The fifth kind of intimacy is like the final coat of gloss we put on our nails after polishing them: It's what makes the color pop instead of being dull. I'm talking about **spiritual intimacy**—which, by the way, has nothing to do with religion. It's the joy of believing, absolutely, that you are in the right place, doing the right thing, with the right person—that you, they, your families, and *the world around you* are better for it. You'll see how spiritual intimacy can manifest a beautiful sense of harmony in your relationship.

You may notice that vulnerability is part of what makes something intimate. Brené Brown, one of the people I admire most in this world, has taught us so much about that. "We cultivate love when we allow our most vulnerable and powerful selves to be deeply seen and known," Brené says. "The difficult thing is that vulnerability is the first thing I look for in you and the last thing I'm willing to show you. In you, it's courage and daring. In me, it's weakness."

I cannot emphasize enough that vulnerability is *not* weakness. It's the pathway to our soul. Brené speaks to the vital role it plays in relationships: "There is no intimacy without vulnerability."[6]

In a healthy, romantic relationship, all 5 Kinds of Intimacy are braided together, each one a vital strand in keeping the relationship long-lasting, meaningful, and sexy too.

I know, thanks to my own journey from up-tight prude to joyfully romantic woman, that life is a lot happier and healthier when we experience the full range of intimacies. This is why I've made it my mission to help others set sail on their own journeys.

I believe that love really can last forever. I say this despite my having spent years as a divorce lawyer! No, that's not right; I say it *because* of the years I spent as a divorce lawyer. Divorce court is full of examples of the ways relationships *don't* work—but every one of them can offer a lesson in how things might have gone differently.

> In a healthy, romantic relationship, all 5 Kinds of Intimacy are braided together, each one a vital strand in keeping the relationship long-lasting, meaningful, and sexy too.

---

[6] "Brené Brown," https://brenebrown.com/.

Love Goggles

Way before couples wind up in divorce court, they fall blissfully in love. Oh, the joy! Love is truly divine. It's exhilarating, for goodness' sake! We're giddy, excited; our body tingles while our brain is awash in happy hormones. Love makes us feel alive. Rose-tinted glasses are nothing compared to love goggles.

The problem is that sooner or later, the love goggles get lost. Suddenly we're back in the real world—*ouch!* It can be quite a surprise. But hey, if given a chance, we'd do it all over again. Who cares about future clarity when you can be lost in a loving fog, right?

> This book is for you if you want the most happiness possible from your romantic relationship.

Well, actually . . . I do! I love the intensity of love. However, that's not all I want for you. I want you to also have clarity. I don't want your blissful love to die a long, slow miserable death. I want you to stay in love! I want you to use this book to help you see through your love goggles so you can decide how well your relationship aligns with what you really want.

If you discover that you're only getting a small percentage of the recommended dose of intimacy, I hope you'll use your euphoria to add more intimacy, *pronto*. If that's not possible, you might want to consider moving on sooner rather than later. Take it from me, love is plentiful when you're skilled at intimacy.

In this book, I'm going to give you the tools you'll need when your love goggles come off. This way, with the help of your partner, you'll be able to create the necessary intimacy that will guarantee a life filled with love and laughter.

Is This Book for You?

This book is for you if you want the most happiness possible from your romantic relationship. This book is for you if you believe in true love. It's for you if you're looking for a partner—or if you have a partner you want to keep, even if you've been drifting apart.

> Human beings are designed—programmed, if you will—to seek out relationships. We are all made for love.

No matter your relationship status, you deserve love, intimacy, and joy. In this book, I'm going to teach you what you need to know to get it.

Human beings are designed—programmed, if you will—to seek out relationships. We are all made for love. No matter what you've been through, I believe *you* have the capacity for a loving relationship that lights you up, sparking a delicious fire in your body, mind, and soul.

That's why I'm going to teach you about the five kinds of intimacy. They're exactly what you need to keep your love alive.

That's why I wrote this book. For you.

PART ONE

What You Need to Know About Intimacy

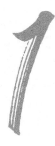

What the Heck Is Intimacy Anyway?

Mary and Brendan were still "best friends" when they filed for divorce. So much so that even the people who knew them best were completely shocked to receive the news. From the outside, their relationship looked perfect.

"*Why?*" everyone kept asking them.

The only answer they ever gave was, "We love each other, but we aren't in love with each other anymore."

Despite all their love, they thought there was no way they would be able to recover what they felt they'd lost—so, sadly, the two of them went their separate ways.

Recently, Brendan came to one of my workshops, where he learned about the 5 Kinds of Intimacy. He came up to me afterward, looking truly forlorn.

"If my wife and I had known about this back then," he said, shaking his head, "we might never have gotten divorced."

Brendan's story is not unusual—especially the way it ended. Personally, I think our national divorce rate should be all the indication

1

we need that we are failing miserably at the fundamental premise of a happy life.

You've probably heard that close to half of marriages end in divorce. What are we doing wrong that the path of love leads to this for almost half the couples out there?

Are you ready to hear the brutal truth?

Love ISN'T everything.

Love ISN'T all you need.

I know it's contrary to everything you've learned (or sung) since you were a kid, but it's true. A marriage[7] requires more than just love to be fulfilling. It needs substance. If you've read the title of this book, you can probably guess what that substance is.

Intimacy.

Our culture frequently equates love with intimacy, sometimes using these terms interchangeably. But they're very different. It's incredibly important to clarify things if we want to be able to create, repair, and maintain a happy, healthy love.

Love, lust, or infatuation is often what draws us to someone, fueling a desire to connect with them. It's our enjoyment of that connection that drives us to commit to our relationship in the hope that our pleasure will continue as well. Somewhere down the line, much to our chagrin, we realize that neither the relationship nor the love is satisfying us any- 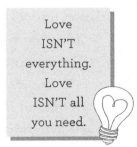 more. We have a craving but can't figure out what will satisfy it.

This is often the point at which people have affairs. If we're lucky, we wake up to the fact that what we crave is intimacy *before* we "fall in love" with someone other than our partner. Think of intimacy like protein. By itself, it's filling but not necessarily tasty. But when it's paired

Love ISN'T everything. Love ISN'T all you need.

---

[7] For the purposes of this book, I use the term *marriage* as a form of shorthand for a long-term, committed romantic relationship, regardless of legality.

with love, it can be fulfilling *and* delicious. It will satisfy your hunger yet also whet your appetite in anticipation of future delights.

"That's all fine and good, Beth," you may be saying, "but what the hell *is* intimacy?"

I'm so glad you asked.

The Hardest Question You've Never Been Asked

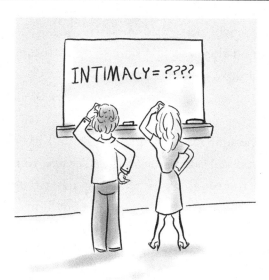

Before I tell you what intimacy means to me, I want you to take a moment to try to answer that question yourself.

What is intimacy?

Got your answer? No?

If you're having trouble, rest assured that you are not alone. We have no shortage of confusion about intimacy. Everyone wants it, and we're all trying to find it—but nobody can agree on what it actually is!

When I ask this question, people give all sorts of answers, most of which don't hold up to much scrutiny once you start delving deeper.

But what's most surprising to me is that this is true even for the most renowned relationship experts. They talk about intimacy, but until now, no one's actually come up with a clear, workable understanding or definition of intimacy.

In my workshops, I let the whole group try to find their way to a definition they can agree on. Often, it begins with someone saying, "Intimacy? That's just a polite way to say *sex*, right?"

The group laughs because they're all a little nervous.

Then someone whispers, "Closeness?"

The group nods because this sounds right. Intimacy exists when two people are close.

But then someone asks, "Do you mean *physically* close? Or emotionally close?"

Now everyone squirms in their seats. "Both! Either?"

"Is it when you feel safe with someone because you trust them?"

Everyone in the room begins thinking about their own relationships. The times they had sex with someone but didn't feel much emotional connection—was that "intimate"? What about the opposite? Those deep emotional connections that didn't involve sex at all—were those "intimate"? How about that deep, head-over-heels love you felt for your junior high crush? The two of you never kissed and you barely ever spoke—but somehow you still think about that person, delighting in the powerful rush of romance you felt. Was that intimate?

Someone else asks, "What about a roommate? Are we intimate with our roommate?"

Some of you may be thinking, *Beth, I had all kinds of intimacies with my roommate. One night we both drank too much wine and started playing naked Twister!*

Okay . . . but what about the other kind of roommates? The ones you live with for years, who see you first thing in the morning, who see you when you're sick, who are there during your grocery runs, throughout your TV binges, or after your disastrous dates? You cook meals together. You tell each other secrets. You know each other's family; I mean, you practically *are* each other's family! You don't have sex with each other, but there's no doubt that this is a really deep, important relationship in your life.

Can friendship be "intimate"?

Clearly, intimacy is very hard to define! If you can't define it, how are you supposed to achieve it? If you can't identify what it is, how are you supposed to make sure you're experiencing it? How can you tell if you have as much of it as you need? How are you supposed to get it back, once you feel you've lost it, if you can't even quite explain what "it" is?

These questions can cause anyone to throw up their hands in despair. Fortunately, I'm about to make it much easier for you by removing the vagueness around intimacy. To do that, let's take a look at some of the most common myths I see in my work with clients. To understand what I believe intimacy *is,* it helps to start with what it *isn't.*

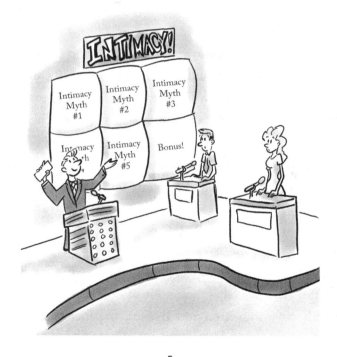

Myths About Intimacy

Intimacy only matters in romantic relationships.
FALSE! We share many kinds of intimacy with many kinds of people. Understanding intimacy will help you navigate all of your relationships.

All intimacy is sexual.
FALSE! You don't have to have sex with someone to be intimate with them. Healthy relationships require five kinds of intimacy; each is equally important. Later in the book, we will dive into examples of sexual intimacy that are sans sex!

Intimacy is always positive.
FALSE! Intimacy doesn't always make us feel good; sometimes it's uncomfortable, painful, or absolutely torturous. In fact, when loved ones push each other's buttons during a fight, what they're doing is using emotional intimacy to wound instead of soothe.

Intimacy always works both ways.
FALSE! We can have intimacy with someone who doesn't have intimacy with us. Peeping Toms take advantage of this form of intimacy. We often experience it while watching live TV. When Will Smith marched onstage at the 2022 Oscars to slap Chris Rock, we shared a very emotionally intimate moment with him. But at the same time, he had no awareness of us on a personal level, so while he probably feels publicly exposed, he doesn't feel intimate with each of us the way we do with him.

Being intimate is our choice.
FALSE! While there are times when we can decide to open up to people or to keep our distance, there are a lot of other times when intimacy occurs whether we like it or not. In fact, the kicker is when people

shut down in order to avoid intimacy, they can inadvertently reveal a lot about themselves, such as their fears, insecurities, or feelings about someone. The irony is that an astute observer can often see exactly what they are trying to hide—which creates intimacy. Crazy, right? But it's true. It's why some people are nervous around therapists and others who are trained in the area of emotional intimacy.

The Sad Tale of Intimacy: Abused and Overused

These days, people use the word *intimacy* as an ambiguous catchall term. We see it often—in self-help books, internet listicles, and magazine articles with titles such as "10 Surefire Ways to Enjoy Intimacy with Your Partner."

But when intimacy remains in the realm of ambiguous generalities, it doesn't particularly help us because we don't really know what it is. We casually throw it out there as something we aspire to have in our relationships. But that isn't specific enough.

In this book, I want to be very, very, *very* specific about intimacy. Whether or not we like it, whether or not we think it is a "positive" or a "negative," intimacy is an important element of our lives. You can have relationships without intimacy—but you can also have intimacy without relationships. For example, you have physical intimacy with the guy you're pressed up against on the subway. You create emotional intimacy with the people at the airport who see you burst into tears when you miss an important flight.

Most of us will experience countless moments of "forced" intimacy like this throughout our lives. We don't choose it. We don't necessarily want it. But it's intimacy all the same.

I'm clearly not the only expert talking about intimacy. But I promise you I'll give you the real deal, the truth about what intimacy is and how to create it. I'll be specific instead of relying on smoke and mirrors. In fact, what makes my approach so impactful is that it's concise, practical, workable, and even measurable. No more running in circles not knowing what's needed for a loving, lasting, fulfilling relationship!

I've waited years to write this book because I needed to prove to myself that this theory works—repeatedly. Consistently. I've invited other relationship experts with decades of experience to challenge me at every step of the way; none have found a reason to dispute it. I'm not a scientific researcher, so I can't show you formal studies, but informally I've seen thousands of people transform their relationship based on what I'm about to teach you.

Starting from scratch to achieve an understanding of what intimacy is and isn't will have a *huge* impact on your relationship. I've seen it over and over again. When a couple focuses on deepening each kind of intimacy in their relationship, something magical happens. Lightning strikes.

And, I should add, it's the *good* kind of lightning! The kind that fills your life with energetic brilliance—keeping your love alive.

Finally, a Working Definition!

When a word is confusing, I do what any word nerd would do: I turn to a dictionary.

> **in·ti·ma·cy** / ˈintəməsē /
> n. (pl. -cies)
> close familiarity or friendship; closeness: *the intimacy between a husband and wife.*
> • a private cozy atmosphere: *the room had a peaceful sense of intimacy about it.*
> • an intimate act, esp. sexual intercourse.
> • an intimate remark: *here she was sitting swapping intimacies with a stranger.*
> • [in sing.] closeness of observation or knowledge of a subject: *he acquired an intimacy with Swahili literature.*

Crazy, right? Looks like the dictionary can't decide on a single definition of the word *intimacy* either!

This gets to the heart of the problem: When we talk about intimacy, we're sometimes talking about completely different things. While one person says "I'm intimate with him" to mean they feel "cozy," someone else uses the same phrase to mean "We're having sex." A third person might be claiming to have expert knowledge. "I have an intimate knowledge of baseball," says your friend in Chicago, but you're pretty sure he's not sleeping with all the Cubs.

This brings me, at long last, to *my* definition of intimacy as it relates to relationships:

Intimacy is a state that results from a connection, closeness, familiarity, exposure, or proximity that is highly personal, so much so that it is likely to cause a feeling of vulnerability.

It's that simple.

Brené Brown offers some brilliant insight on vulnerability. "Vulnerability is not winning or losing," she says. "It's having the courage to show up and be seen when we have no control over the outcome. Vulnerability is not weakness; it's our greatest measure of courage . . . People who wade into discomfort and vulnerability and tell the truth about their stories are the real badasses."[8]

> Intimacy is a state that results from a connection, closeness, familiarity, exposure, or proximity that is highly personal, so much so that it is likely to cause a feeling of vulnerability.

The way we respond to that discomfort, that vulnerability, is highly subjective. It can be good or bad. That's true whether or not we're in a relationship. One person might feel just fine about being pressed up against people on

---

[8] Brené Brown, *Rising Strong: The Reckoning. The Rumble. The Revolution.* (Random House, August 25, 2015), https://www.amazon.com/Rising-Strong-Reckoning-Rumble-Revolution/dp/0812995821/.

the subway, while that same degree of closeness makes another person extremely uncomfortable. Either way, there's vulnerability.

When it comes to relationships, we crave closeness in different ways—and they all matter. It was this insight that led me to recognize the five particular kinds of intimacy.

I realized that love is ephemeral unless substance is provided to maintain and grow it. It's easy for some people to say (and feel) love, but if the feelings aren't accompanied by substance, the love dissipates. I see couples all the time who profess great love for each other, believing that's enough to keep them happy together. But that's as foolish as thinking that enjoying the smell of a good meal is enough to satisfy your hunger.

"I love you so much!" they tell each other. "Isn't that enough?"

Nope. Without substance (intimacy), love is empty. It's like cotton candy: sweet and pretty but unfulfilling.

This is exactly why I developed not just a *theory* of intimacy but also a full-bodied, whole-hearted practice packed with practices, tips, and tools for creating the kind of intimacies in your romantic relationship that bring you true joy and connection. When you add these to love, you'll have a substantive, fulfilling, sexy, loving relationship in which *both partners are satisfied.*

You've Got Options!

If you read my first book, you'll recognize this refrain: People don't know what their options are. No one talks about this stuff! And because no one talks about it, people don't understand what they're missing or why their relationship isn't working.

When it comes to intimacy, a couple might be doing a great job in three or even four of the intimacies. Based on their success in those areas, they think they should be happy, yet there's a nagging feeling that there's got to be more, even though they haven't got a clue what "more" is. Or maybe one partner is happy with the level (or lack) of intimacy, but the other is starved for more.

There are endless examples of people settling for less-than-fulfilling relationships. Sometimes, they don't see the bigger picture, so they don't even know they're settling. Without the bigger picture, how can they possibly know what the possibilities are?

I want you to be aware of how good your relationship could be. Because, quite frankly, if you read this book with a willing partner, it's not that hard to fill your love with the kind of intimacy that turns love into a delicious, healthy meal that leaves you smiling.

To make this as easy as possible for you, Part One of this book is exactly what you need to know about intimacy. I know that it's a lot to take in. That's why at the end of each chapter, you'll find Tantalizing Takeaways: key info you should remember from each chapter, and in some cases, the takeaways are things you'll want to talk to your partner about. (E-books are cool but sharing a print copy with your partner so you can both write in it might be worthwhile. It's especially fun if you each use a different ink color.)

In Part Two, you'll discover a variety of simple, fun, and extremely helpful intimacy practices that will create lots of joyful, fulfilling intimacy.

Think of this as the start of a great adventure. You're about to embark on an exciting journey full of pleasurable discoveries that lead to a lifetime of passionate love. The result is nothing short of transformative.

> Think of this as the start of a great adventure. You're about to embark on an exciting journey full of pleasurable discoveries that lead to a lifetime of passionate love. The result is nothing short of transformative.

Are you a little scared about this adventure? Join the club! Which is why we're going to specifically address the almost universal fear of intimacy next. It may seem like a contradiction, but fear of intimacy is actually completely rational. Ironically, that fear is a sign of how important intimacy is to you. To each of us. We crave, need, and fear intimacy in fairly equal measure.

Tantalizing Takeaways

- It's unreasonable to expect anyone to succeed at marriage without understanding what's required for a happy, healthy, fulfilling long-term relationship.
- Intimacy provides the substance love needs to survive and thrive.
- Each of the 5 Kinds of Intimacy is distinct and vital to relationships; none can substitute for another long term.

2

Fear of Intimacy

I ntimacy can be terrifying.
Justifiably so.

In fact, fear of intimacy may be one of the few characteristics shared by all animals.

Sure, scientists have given fancy names to the various innate defense mechanisms found in different species: camouflage, quills, loud growls, stinky fluids. But at the core, aren't all of these just ways to protect these animals from unwanted intimacy?

When it comes to us humans, we like to pretend that we aren't animals, but that's a foolish notion. Humans can be warm, loving, nurturing beings, but we can also be predatory, manipulative, and aggressive. If we didn't have an innate fear of intimacy, if we walked around allowing everyone to see our weaknesses, insecurities, and blind spots, we'd be easy targets for those with nefarious agendas.

Of course, it's easy to say we should be afraid of intimacy with strangers. But once we're in a relationship, shouldn't our defenses naturally relax?

Well, that would be lovely, but let's think about it more carefully. Let's start at the beginning—or close to it, anyway. Let's imagine a five-year-old child, Kam, who's just starting kindergarten.

The Fear of Rejection—a.k.a. the Fear of Lost Love

Kam has loving parents who treat him well. In turn, Kam adores, respects, and wants to please them. In fact, Kam is so concerned with what his parents think that when he gets in trouble at school for the first time, he's terrified. His teacher sends him home with a note for his parents, but he's too scared to show it to them, so he hides it. He doesn't let them know what happened—not just because he is afraid of being punished but also because he's afraid of disappointing them.

Although Kam's experience with his parents has generally been positive, they did impose a long time-out (ten minutes of isolation, which felt like complete rejection) after he (accidentally) broke an expensive vase a few months ago. Kam knows that getting in trouble at school is even worse than breaking a vase, which makes him worry that if his parents discover that he isn't the "good boy" they expect him to be, they'll withdraw not only their approval but also their love.

Kam isn't really worried about survival (he believes his parents will probably still feed him, though he's not sure since this has never happened before); what he fears is rejection. As a human being, Kam is biologically wired to seek belonging and connection, so much so that he's programmed to instinctively fear rejection. Interestingly, rejection is as painful to humans as *physical* pain.

Let that sink in for a moment.

All of us are programmed to protect ourselves from rejection in the same way we are programmed to protect ourselves from physical pain.

Have you ever heard of a kid deliberately touching a hot stove on more than one occasion?

Me neither.

The greater the pain, the faster we learn.

That's why rejection hurts so much. That's why we work so hard to avoid it, especially when it comes from those who matter most. The stakes are highest when we are most invested.

No wonder we're afraid of intimacy.

Kam isn't being irrational when he decides to hide the note from his teacher; it's no different from the resistance of a trapped animal when a caring person tries to help it. It's our natural instinct to protect ourselves from risk.

Do you see the irony? We have a natural instinct to protect ourselves from risk, but that instinct coexists with a deeply wired need for intimate connection. That's a scientific Catch-22.

Why We Need Each Other: The Science of Intimacy

Throughout thousands of years of evolution, people who could maintain close relationships with others were more likely to survive.

That's especially true for physical intimacy, which in some ways is the easiest kind to describe since it's right there on the surface. When you are in close contact with a person you trust, when you hug or hold hands or touch, your body chemistry changes. Your brain surges with oxytocin, the "love hormone," which in turn triggers the release of other "happy hormones," dopamine and serotonin, making you feel better, happier, even safer. Levels of your "stress hormone," cortisol, decline, making your heart rate and blood pressure drop as well. In short, human contact doesn't just make you feel better; it also—literally—makes you healthier.[9]

> Rejection hurts so much. That's why we work so hard to avoid it, especially when it comes from those who matter most. The stakes are highest when we are most invested.

The opposite is true too. Being apart from people doesn't simply *feel* bad; it *is* bad. People who spend too much time alone are at increased

---

[9] Taylor Mallory Holland, "Facts About Touch: How Human Contact Affects Your Health and Relationships," Dignity Health | Facts About Touch, April 28, 2018, https://www.dignityhealth.org/articles/facts-about-touch-how-human-contact-affects-your-health-and-relationships.

risk for hypertension, cardiovascular disease, dementia, immune system dysfunction, and depression.[10]

We evolved as social creatures. Our very survival as a species has always depended on close relationships with other people who could keep us safe from danger. Our biochemistry reflects this fact.

Loneliness puts the body into a long-term state of "fight or flight," the acute distress response that an animal experiences when its life is threatened. This has a profound impact on our physical and mental health. One reason breakups hurt is that your body is sending you a warning sign: being alone is dangerous!

Our bodies aren't wrong. Even now, when we're safe from cave bears and saber-toothed tigers, being alone is still dangerous. It's as detrimental to our long-term health as if we were obese or smoked fifteen cigarettes a day![11] Because of the toll loneliness takes on the body, people in intimate relationships will live, on average, two years longer than single people.[12]

You see the irony, right? The data is clear: We need intimacy. Yet so often when we have the opportunity for intimacy, when we face the tremendous risk of being vulnerable with another person, we run like hell in the other direction.

I've seen so much avoidance that I'm almost shocked when people *have* successfully learned how to integrate a healthy amount of intimacy

---

[10] Matt Reynolds, "The Weird Science of Loneliness and Our Brains," Wired (Conde Nast, March 30, 2021), https://www.wired.com/story/weird-science-of-loneliness-brains/.

[11] Sophia Ktori, "Scientists Show What Loneliness Looks Like in the Brain," GEN, December 16, 2020, https://www.genengnews.com/news/scientists-show-what-loneliness-looks-like-in-the-brain/.

[12] Haomiao Jia and Erica I. Lubetkin, "Life Expectancy and Active Life Expectancy by Marital Status among Older U.S. Adults," National Center for Biotechnology Information, August 15, 2020, https://www.ncbi.nlm.nih.gov/pmc/articles/PMC7452000/.

into their life. This is something that requires dedication, risk-taking, and a whole lotta practice.

Heck, I've bungee jumped in New Zealand, skydived, and driven race cars at 150 miles per hour, but despite everything I know about intimacy, none of these things scares me as much as falling in love. In truth, most of us are much more scared of broken hearts than we are of broken bones.

How do we address this deep-seated fear? How do we challenge it so that our relationships are not constantly fraught with fear of rejection? How do we face down our fear of intimacy so we don't ruin our chances for the deep love, joy, and pleasure we deserve?

The starting place might not be where you expect because the work doesn't actually begin in our partnerships; it begins a little closer to home. To face your fear of intimacy, you must first tell the truth to the most important person in your life. Even if that person is the harshest, scariest, meanest person in your life.

It's Scary to Expose Yourself . . . to Yourself

You know who most people are most afraid of intimacy with?

Themselves.

Yep.

It all starts with being intimate with yourself.

Let's imagine that Kam (from the prior chapter) has grown up, but age hasn't rid him of his fear of disappointing his loved ones. These days though, instead of having trouble at school, Kam has started day drinking—so much so that people at work have expressed concern.

Kam's angry that they are "butting into his life." He's also scared and confused about what to do.

Do you think Kam is going to be willing to talk to his spouse about his colleagues' concerns? Do you think he's capable of that level of voluntary emotional intimacy? Or do you think he's more likely to spend his drive home making excuses to himself about how his day drinking isn't a problem, so he doesn't need to mention it to his spouse?

When we fool ourselves or avoid facing the issues we aren't comfortable with, it's because we have a lack of emotional intimacy with ourselves. We don't see, know, or understand ourselves because we are actively hiding, repressing, or refusing to acknowledge the things with which we are less than thrilled.

Here are some examples of ways people exhibit a lack of self-intimacy:

- Refusing to look at themselves naked in a mirror
- Ignoring self-destructive actions, such as drinking, taking drugs, or partaking in dangerous activities
- Frequently blaming others for their own unhappiness
- Constantly feeling that everything happens *to* them instead of acknowledging their contribution to situations
- Comparing themselves to others and/or putting others down (openly or not)
- Repeatedly leaving jobs, marriages, or friendships because no one "gets" them

Take a Good Look

Wonder what an emotionally self-intimate person might do in Kam's situation?

They'd probably give careful consideration to the people who expressed concern. Are their colleagues true friends, or are they acquaintances trying to stir up trouble? Either way, they'd challenge themself to decide whether any part of what their colleagues said rings true, even in the deepest part of their gut.

They might even apply logic, acknowledging that if there's no truth to what their colleagues said, there wouldn't be much harm in sharing it with their partner. They'd recognize that their urge to keep it a secret might indicate a problem.

When we withhold from ourselves (or from our partner) who we are, what we want, or what we desire, it's a negative reflection on the level of emotional intimacy in the relationship. From there, it's not uncommon to turn our discomfort into resentment as justification for avoiding intimacy. Instead of accepting that we aren't handling things well, we tell ourselves, "I'm only afraid to share this because my partner is so judgmental" or "I can't tell them because they won't understand."

Again, think of five-year-old Kam, terrified that his parents will be disappointed but not giving them the opportunity to prove him wrong.

These are real fears. You are allowed to feel them. Most people do. As you read this book, I only urge you to not let fear win. I say that as someone who let the fear win for a very long time.

When I got divorced after staying in my unhappy marriage for twenty-three years, I was determined to start living my life differently. I felt like I'd been walking around with toilet paper hanging from my skirt for all those years; everyone else saw it—but I had no idea! I had been deliberately blind because I felt hopeless. Seeing myself was so depressing that I simply stopped looking.

When I finally felt empowered enough to get divorced, I vowed to stop looking away when I saw things I didn't like about myself. I swore I would stop pretending to be okay with things that actually made me feel bad. I finally realized that if I could be brave enough to see myself, I'd be strong enough to make improvements.

Lack of intimacy with yourself can feel like looking at yourself through an Instagram filter while pretending it's real. Believe me, no matter how flawed you are, you deserve so much more.

In the words of the inimitable Maya Angelou, "I don't trust people who don't love themselves and yet tell me, 'I love you.' There is an

African saying which is: Be careful when a naked person offers you a shirt."[13]

So, let's get you a shirt, shall we?

How to Be Intimate with Your One and Only

If you're like most people today, you'll have more than one romantic relationship in your lifetime. Some might be fleeting, a week of erotic passion you will never forget. Other relationships might last for decades, till death do you part. Maybe you'll kiss a hundred people . . . or a very lucky three. There is no wrong number.

But here's the deal: you only ever have one relationship with yourself.

That's why it kills me that I stayed mired in fear until I was in my mid-forties. Worse yet, so many people stay mired in fear their entire lives. It pains me that they'll live out their days without ever truly experiencing the joy, pleasure, and self-acceptance that can come with deep self-intimacy.

Let's take a quick look at how self-intimacy, or a lack of it, can affect us in each of the five areas:

Physical intimacy is a huge problem for many of us. Some of us hate our bodies so much that we avoid looking at or touching them any more than is absolutely necessary. For some, their discomfort is limited to certain parts of their body, but I know women who refuse to even glance at a mirror because they're so convinced they are ugly or fat. (Trust me: I've been there before.) The problem is if we're not comfortable loving our own body, how are we going to be comfortable using our body to love our partner?

Think about all the people who have had health issues or surgeries, including women who've had mastectomies and men who can't get

---

[13] "Maya Angelou Quotes: 15 of the Best," The Guardian (Guardian News and Media, May 29, 2014), https://www.theguardian.com/books/2014/may/28/maya-angelou-in-fifteen-quotes

erections. It's all painfully difficult, so it's not surprising that it starts eroding our confidence, making it tempting to disassociate from our physical selves rather than face our issues.

Yet, in the words of Carl Jung, "Until you make the unconscious conscious, it will direct your life and you will call it fate."

What if you imagine having a different relationship with your body? A relationship in which you could look in the mirror and feel something other than disappointment or disgust? What if you could feel contentment? Pride? Maybe even a little *pleasure?*

A healthy level of physical self-intimacy would include awareness as a substitute for avoidance. Instead of ignoring it, you'd be willing to love it. You'd get to know it so that you could care for it better; you'd probably even want to touch yourself. After all, we humans enjoy touching what we love. (I don't just mean touching in a sexual way. I also mean touching in other ways, like stroking your shoulder or rubbing your hands or whatever.)

Wouldn't that be something? To feel *good* when you touch your own body?

As for **emotional intimacy**, we live in a world full of people who truly have no idea as to who they are or what they really want. They can't admit to themselves what they're afraid of—or what they're not good at. Sometimes they conceal this fact with bravado, arrogance, or narcissism, but it's only because they're not emotionally intimate with themselves. They might be in constant pursuit of fame, money, or beauty, pretending that those things equate to happiness. They continue to allow their subconscious to dictate their behavior, so they never learn to overcome the issues that hold them back, which ensures they will never get what they actually want.

> Emotional intimacy, we live in a world full of people who truly have no idea as to who they are or what they really want.

But why not allow yourself to imagine a future in which you choose something different? One in which instead of avoiding certain truths about yourself, you invite them in and learn from them? What would happen if you were to face the truths that you don't like and then change them? How would things shift in your life and your relationships if you were to give yourself permission to get to know yourself and then allow yourself to bring forth your whole self in your relationship?

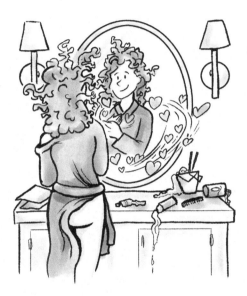

Take a moment here and close your eyes. Allow yourself to envision a version of your life in which you know exactly who you are, what you're brilliant at, and what you want—one in which you truly *love* your perfectly imperfect self! Imagine the confidence you'd have if you were to love yourself as you are right now! You may not know it, but I swear it's possible. Even for you. For each of us.

Almost all of us have some hang-ups when it comes to **sexual intimacy,** but the most prevalent ones relate to masturbation. There are countless people who have been taught that self-pleasure is wrong or that there are only certain circumstances in which it's acceptable. These beliefs can't help but spill over into their sexual relationships, creating a lack of insight into their own pleasure, resistance to exploring new things, or an inability to express their needs. Over time, these problems can erode all pleasure, passion, and laughter.

With self-intimacy comes freedom. The truth is, loving yourself makes it much more likely that you'll be able to love your partner better. It also makes it easier for you to receive sexy love in return. Wouldn't it be amazing if love included delicious, mind-blowing, skin-tingling sexual pleasure? How exciting would that be?

In each of these kinds of intimacy—physical, emotional, and sexual—a lack of self-intimacy can rob you of the ability to be intimate with your partner.

To illustrate the remaining two kinds of intimacy, I'm going to tell you a story.

One night, not so long ago, I was sitting on a quiet beach in Cancún, Mexico. I was all by myself. Just me in my chair, right where the waves curled into the sand, enjoying the thousands of stars shining brightly. I was wearing a short sundress, savoring the cool breeze against my skin over most of my body. It was delicious. It was bliss. It was sexy. It was kind of a turn-on.

I was so happy, even proud, to be alone, having created this opportunity for myself. I wasn't wishing for a companion. I was deliberately doing exactly what I wanted. I had arranged this as a solo beach vacation not because I didn't have anyone to travel with but because I wanted time alone to indulge my desire for some "blue therapy."[14] I felt powerful. Wonderful. Romantic.

---

[14] The gentle movement of water lapping, the sound of the waves, the salty air . . . Spending time in a natural environment featuring a body of water has many benefits for our health and well-being. And this practice even has a name: "blue therapy." https://www.lifestyleasia.com/bk/living/wellness/what-is-blue-therapy-mental-health/amp/.

Yes, romantic. I didn't need a partner to enjoy **romantic intimacy**.

Better still, I luxuriated in the **spiritual intimacy** of the moment as well.

I was 100 percent glad to be there, with everything exactly as it was. I didn't feel guilty that someone or something else needed me elsewhere. I wasn't depriving anybody of anything. I wasn't breaking any law by being on the beach at night. I wasn't being defensive by trying to prove that I could be happy on my own. I simply was happy. All was okay. It was *better* than okay. It was "right."

At its core, that's what spiritual intimacy is: a sense of rightness.

My hope for you is that after reading this book, you'll allow yourself to live a life overflowing with intimacy that fills you with joy. That you'll give yourself the freedom to enjoy *all 5 kinds of intimacy* with yourself—and with anyone you choose.

In the next chapter, we'll look at some of the obstacles that make intimacy difficult and learn how to face them head-on.

But first, I have something to confess.

> My hope for you is that after reading this book, you'll allow yourself to live a life overflowing with intimacy that fills you with joy. That you'll give yourself the freedom to enjoy *all five kinds of intimacy* with yourself—and with anyone you choose.

Tantalizing Takeaways

- Humans are programmed to both seek and avoid intimacy.
- Facing your fear of intimacy starts with . . . you. How comfortable are you with acknowledging, accepting, and loving your less than perfect parts?
- Becoming more intimate with yourself will allow you to exercise more conscious awareness when deciding to embrace or avoid intimacy with others.

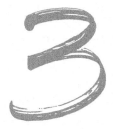

Intimacy Doesn't Have
to Be So Hard

Here's my confession:

I spent a couple of years unsure of how to explain intimacy to my clients. This, even as a relationship coach who reads almost fanatically to keep up with all the latest research! If I couldn't *explain* intimacy, despite learning from all the other experts, how could my clients understand it? I drove myself nuts trying to come up with a workable framework to make it easier for my clients.

To be fair, that's not to say I didn't have some half-decent ideas. I mean, I'm smart and well-read. But more than anything, the early seeds of this book came from my clients.

When people came into my shop, attended my workshops, or hired me as their coach, I began to notice some common refrains:

> *"My partner wants more sex; I want more emotional connection."*

> *"Even though we still have lots of sex, we're not as close as we used to be. No matter how often we talk about it, we can't figure out why."*

25

"I love them, but I'm not in love with them anymore."

"I wish they would initiate sex sometimes instead of making me ask, only to be rejected."

I hated this. I'm a problem-solver. I wanted to teach my clients not only how to fix things *now* but also how to course-correct next time life knocks them off track ('cause we all know it will!). It wasn't enough for them to just start having more conversations or better sexy fun; those are just temporary fixes. They needed to understand *why* those things matter in order to cure the underlying issues, not just minimize the symptoms.

Yet even when I had clarity about the fundamental cause of their problems, my clients were perplexed by my diagnosis: "You're both intimacy-deprived." Sometimes they even became argumentative, protesting, "No, it's just that she wants too much sex," or "It's just because he never listens to me," or "I'm simply bored in the bedroom," or "It just feels like we're not connecting as deeply as I'd hoped."

After all, have you ever said to yourself, "Dang, I need a big dose of intimacy today"? If you have, you might just be my new hero!

Let's face it: How could you know you want it when no one ever taught you *what it is,* let alone why it makes life better? It's no different than when I went to my doctor, complaining of hair loss and asking for a medicated shampoo to fix the problem. I had no idea that what I *needed* was thyroid medication because that was the underlying cause of my problem.

Of course, most relationship experts agree that people want and need intimacy. I wasn't unique in focusing on it—but I was unique in my approach. I was compelled to thoroughly understand, clarify, define, and categorize intimacy.

In other words, I took a lawyer-like approach to the topic.

Consider this book my appellate brief, within which I will attempt to prove that the 5 Kinds of Intimacy—physical, emotional, sexual, romantic, and spiritual—are what all happy, healthy marriages rely on.

That being said, I actually want you to enjoy reading this book, so I promise you it's not written like a lawyer's brief! Also, just because it was hard for me to create this new paradigm for lasting love doesn't mean it has to be hard for you to implement it. In fact, one of the reasons I've spent months torturing myself by writing this book is because this approach to intimacy is not only theoretically sound, it's also simple to implement. If it were complicated, I would have assumed no one would do it, so I'd have gone back to the beach! The fact that it's effective and easy is what convinced me that everyone should have a chance to use it.

> None of the 5 Kinds of Intimacy is more innately valuable than any other.

We've Tried Before, but Nothing Changed

Part of the reason intimacy has felt so impossible to attain is because the lack of specificity made it similar to chasing a moving target. If we believed intimacy was sex, then why did we feel unsatisfied afterward? If intimacy was about emotional connection, why did people have affairs despite claiming their spouses were their best friends? No matter what we did, we couldn't "catch" intimacy.

That's no longer true. You're going to have a thorough understanding of what intimacy is, so you'll have no trouble recognizing it in the future. You'll know what's needed to create a fulfilling relationship. You won't ever be confused about what kind of intimacy you have or lack.

Another reason intimacy might have felt so elusive is that you were craving one kind of intimacy while your partner was longing for another. You might have been like so many other couples who are stuck because neither is getting what they want, so neither is giving what the other wants. Each is convinced that until they get their needs met, they shouldn't "have to" meet the other's. It's a painful "chicken or the egg" dilemma.

This destructive cycle is frequently exacerbated by a belief that one form of intimacy is better or worse than another. I cannot stress this enough: None of the five kinds of intimacy is more innately valuable than any other. That might surprise you, especially since we have all received some very polarizing messages about what matters most in a loving relationship. In other words, we've been taught there is an unspoken hierarchy.

In truth, our current culture prioritizes emotional intimacy over sexual intimacy. We tend to demean and admonish those who dare complain about a lack of sex while martyring those who complain about a lack of emotional intimacy in their relationship. There's a deeply ingrained imbalance here—one that must be challenged because it is as damaging as it is prevalent.

Once you accept that each of the five intimacies is equally important, you'll find it easier to get unstuck. The advantage to this is that you can start building intimacy in whichever area feels easiest. Your success in that area will not only strengthen your relationship, it will also give you the confidence you need to address the other ones.

You'll also find it freeing to recognize that each kind of intimacy describes a different type of connection. This means that even though you experience one kind of intimacy with someone, you don't automatically have any of the others. Nor does it mean the others will follow. While it's certainly possible to use one intimacy to help create another, it's not a given.

> In truth, our current culture prioritizes emotional intimacy over sexual intimacy. We tend to demean and admonish those who dare complain about a lack of sex while martyring those who complain about a lack of emotional intimacy in their relationship.

As you delve deeper into this book, remember that each kind of intimacy is specifically unique and distinct from the others—even though they sometimes overlap. I know it's tempting to believe that an extra dose of one intimacy can make up for a lack in another, but you'll save yourself a lot of frustration if you believe me when I tell you that you can't substitute one for another long-term.

When you start with love and add all five of these intimacies, you'll wind up with a happy, healthy, passionate relationship that will last. A well-balanced blend of all five is where the magic happens.

So then, why is this delicious blend so hard to come by? Intimacy is free, zero calories, and available to everyone; you'd think we'd all have an abundance of it, right?

As we talked about previously, most of us have some resistance when it comes to voluntarily engaging in some, if not all, of the different kinds of intimacy. Just think of the stereotypical "player" who's happy to hop in the sack with someone they just met but runs for the hills when their closest friend asks about their dying dad.

Relationships struggle when one or more of these intimacies are deficient or out of balance—or when a partner puts more emphasis on one kind than another or wants a deeper level of a particular kind of intimacy than the other person is able or inclined to give.

What You've Learned Can Hurt You

While I'm big into personal responsibility, it's foolish to ignore how our societal norms make things even harder for people. That's not to say I'm in favor of perpetuating the current divisions along gender lines (I'm absolutely *not*!), only that for purposes of improving our chances of happiness, we need to face today's reality, which is this:

Very few women appreciate emotional intimacy through sexual intimacy, and very few men enjoy emotional intimacy when not engaging in sexual intimacy.

Before you scream at me in frustration, I should note this doesn't mean we have to remain stuck in this dynamic for the rest of our lives! Knowledge is power, so you're going to be able to make big changes after reading this book. The goal is for all of us to learn to appreciate each kind of intimacy so we can feel well-loved 24/7, wherever we are. To paraphrase one of my clients, "I can't believe I can feel so much love while fully dressed!"

Bonus Time

Another incentive for you . . . did I mention that big bonuses await you when you enjoy more fulfilling intimacy in your relationship? They really do! In addition to having a relationship that gives you all the good vibes you've always dreamed of, you will also be better able to deal with all sorts of outside forces. Even if you lose your parents, get fired from your job, move across the country, struggle with your kids, or experience any other curveballs life may throw at you, you'll still have a deep well of loving support to draw from.

> Very few women appreciate emotional intimacy through sexual intimacy, and very few men enjoy emotional intimacy when not engaging in sexual intimacy.

Why? Because when your primary relationship is powerfully strong, you inherently absorb some of its strength. It's pretty miraculous—and absolutely true.

So right now, before we go any further, I want you to take a moment to think about how you'd like your relationship to feel—for *your* sake, not anybody else's. What are your deepest desires? What are you hoping to think, feel, and dream when you're with your partner?

Isn't it energizing to think about what you *want* rather than just settling for what you have? It gives me the happy jiggles just thinking about it for you!

Of course, it's not like you can just snap your fingers and make everything better. (I keep wishing, though!) Before you start trying to "fix" things, you have to understand what is and isn't serving you. You have to take stock of where your relationship is currently so you can figure out how to get to where you want to be.

Your Annual Intimacy Review: Coming Soon!

Have you ever wondered why the only place where we receive an annual review is at work? I've yet to meet anyone who provides annual reviews of friendships or romantic relationships.

When you get an annual review at work, you discover what you've done well ("Your client communication is top-notch!") as well as where you've messed up ("Your internal email response time could use some work."). If you've got a good manager handling your review, you'll then work together to create a plan for improvement moving forward.

This is exactly what I think you should do in your relationship after you've finished reading this book. By then, you'll have mastered the fundamental relationship building blocks. While it might feel scary to put your relationship under the microscope, I think it's fair to say that not looking is a lot more dangerous.

I'm giving you a heads-up about this now because I don't want to upset you by surprising you with what could feel like a pop quiz at the end of the book. Plus, my intention isn't to catch you off guard; it's to help inspire you to apply to your own life what you learn throughout the book. I've been guilty of reading books without applying their lessons to my life, and I realize what a waste that was. I'm hoping you'll want to get the most out of this book, which includes bravely completing the State of Your Union assessment that you'll encounter later. Doing so will allow you to celebrate your relationship's strengths and indicate opportunities for improvement. It's obviously up to you, but I really think it's worthwhile.

Slides Aren't Always Fun

I call this book a *guidebook* because my goal is not just to help you *understand* each kind of intimacy but also to help you *create* each one. I'm giving you a framework to clearly evaluate where your relationship is today—right here, right now—so you can immediately get started on improving it. If things are going well now, you might think it's so easy that it won't make a big difference. But take my word—it will. If your relationship is rough right now, it might be harder but imperative. Given that I don't want you to be caught by surprise by an assessment later in this book, you should be darn sure that I don't want you to be caught by surprise when your relationship finally hits rock bottom after years of slowly sliding downhill!

That slide can take place slowly, perhaps slowly enough that you don't even realize it's happening. Or maybe you do realize it, but you're just hoping things are going to get better . . . until the day you wake up to discover it's too late.

The average couple waits. They start out so happy that when they become a little less happy together, they figure it's normal. They can't help feeling a bit cocky; surely, their love is so strong that nothing will wear it down. So they just wait for things to improve "naturally."

But this doesn't happen. As time goes by, the couple might even become indignant: How could this happen to them? They were *sooo* madly in love! This can't be real! The frustration builds up so much that they fight over everything. Each is convinced that if the other would just take the trash out once in a while or stop complaining about how many weekends are spent watching sports, everything would be fine.

After a few years of this, they realize the fighting doesn't help, so they stop. But the issues are still there, getting heavier as they become mired in blame, shame, guilt, and obligation. This cycle generally lasts about six years before someone loses their cool, giving voice to the dreaded "D" word. Only then does one or the other finally suggest they seek professional help.

Wait. Did you catch that?

The average couple is unhappy for an average of six years before they seek professional help to repair their relationship.

Can you imagine driving your car for six years with the check engine light lit up? I'm pretty sure you'd only do that if you assumed there was no saving it.

I think the same applies to a relationship. Which is why I think most couples aren't seeking counseling to repair their marriage. They're seeking permission to call it quits.

Please don't be that couple.

Invest more in your relationship so you can expect more from your relationship.

Get Rid of Hairballs

I often tell my clients that unresolved issues turn into a giant hairball. Think of everything that bugs you but doesn't get resolved as a piece of hair. Some are bigger than others. Some are knotted up; others aren't. You figure that since you don't know what else to do with this hair, you might as well swallow it to avoid having to look at it all the time. This works so well at the beginning that you find yourself swallowing more and more hair. Now you don't have to think about it, right?

> I think most couples aren't seeking counseling to repair their marriage. They're seeking permission to call it quits.

So it works for a while. You swallow this problem, that problem, this little habit that annoys you, that behavior that makes you furious. And you go on like this for a year, two years, five years . . .

The problem? While none of those individual strands of hair were large enough to choke you, the whole mess of them has now gotten so tangled up that it's a giant hairball too big to ignore. It's upsetting your stomach, maybe causing ulcers. You've tried to cough it up or even poop it out, but it's too damn big.

The only way to deal with it is to pull out each and every little piece, one strand at a time (just like it went in!). To avoid swallowing it again, you've got to identify the problem it represents and then resolve it.

It's slow work, but that's okay! Almost all relationships have to do that work at some point. Most have to do it at *many* points. The tremendous advantage you'll now have is that your understanding of intimacy will speed up the process considerably. You'll be able to identify issues lickety-split: "Here's an emotional intimacy issue." "Oh, this right here? It's all about sexual intimacy." You'll have the information you need to understand the problems in your relationship and the tools to resolve them.

When you've finished, not only will you feel better, you'll also be well-equipped to make sure you never again swallow another hair!

Okay, enough about hairballs. Blech!

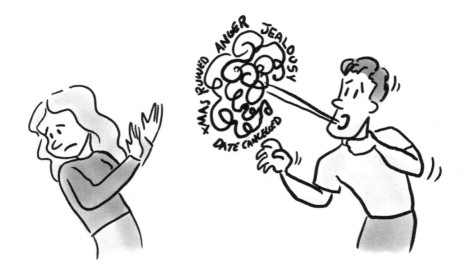

If It's Good Enough for Serena Williams . . .

Do you know what you want in your relationship? I'm looking for specifics rather than vague concepts, like love, security, and respect. How do you want those feelings to be manifested? Are you clear about your priorities?

In other words, what do you need most versus what would you like but can be happy without? Are you getting enough of what you need? Are you getting *any* of what you need?

As the character of Richard Williams says to his kids in *King Richard,* the movie about the remarkable rise of tennis players Serena and Venus Williams, "If you fail to plan, then you plan to fail."

This is no less true for your relationship than it was for the young phenoms' tennis careers.

When we enter relationships without any idea as to what we want, expect, or need from them, it's almost impossible to find happiness. We often start romantic relationships from a very idealistic place: "I'm in love! My partner's amazing! This is everything I've ever wanted!"

That's wonderful. I would never want to deprive you of the starry-eyed, weak-kneed, hot-and-heavy perks of new love. But sometimes, we're mooning over our new sweetheart so intensely that we forget to ask what we want and even what we need.

This book will show you how to be practical about your romantic relationships so that both you and your beloved are happily fulfilled.

Are you ready? Do you believe me when I say it doesn't have to be so hard? Good! Time to explore each kind of intimacy—how it looks, how it feels—and what to do to get more of it in ways that feel good to *you.*

> What do you need most versus what would you like but can be happy without? Are you getting enough of what you need? Are you getting any of what you need?

Tantalizing Takeaways

- It's true—intimacy really isn't *that* complicated or complex. But *fostering* intimacy requires courage.
- Swallowing your problems is a choking hazard! Instead, face them head-on, one at a time, as soon as they crop up.
- Ask yourself: What do I need? What do I want? Am I satisfied or settling? Am I avoiding or ignoring anything about myself or my partner? What does my partner need and want? How can I provide that and more to them?

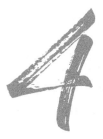

Let's Get Physical

Physical intimacy can include touching—a hug, a hand on the small of the back, a caress on the cheek. But it is also created when someone, even a stranger, invades your personal space via proximity. For example, you experience physical intimacy when squeezed into a crowded elevator or train. In this chapter, we'll cozy up to this kind of intimacy, taking a closer look at how to cultivate awareness and appreciation of physical intimacy in our relationships.

***

That's right: you can experience physical intimacy with people you've never met.

That's not what most people think of when they think of physical intimacy. They assume it's all about "getting physical" in your relationship. The touches, kisses, and sexy stuff you experience with your partner have to be physical intimacy, right?

Absolutely! But that's far from the *only* kind of physical intimacy you experience. Sharing a bed with your lover or sitting at the kitchen table drinking coffee with your spouse are also forms of physical intimacy.

Of all the intimacies, this is the one that we share most often with strangers because the only thing required to establish physical intimacy is proximity. As humans, we are social creatures and with sociability comes physical intimacy.

Once you understand this, it's easy to see that physical intimacy with strangers is a regular occurrence in life, taking place when you're in an elevator, on a bus, on a subway car, or inside a crowded café. It's hard to avoid it, even if we want to.

If you want to get to your meeting on the fortieth floor, you'll probably take the elevator. During the ride, you may be squished up against a bunch of strangers, as if you were sardines, all of you avoiding eye contact as much as possible. Or perhaps there will be just two of you—each leaning against an opposing wall. Either way, you can't help but be physically aware of the other person or people who are inhabiting this space, breathing the same air. It's not necessarily comfortable, but it *is* intimate.

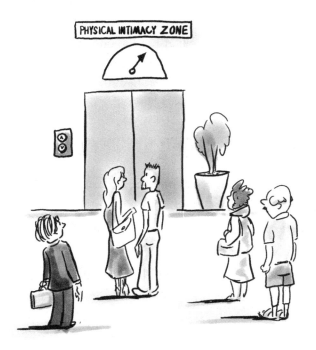

One of the telltale signs of unwanted intimacy is the effort expended by people who are trying to ignore or escape it. When people are thrust into physical intimacy with strangers, they will often shrink into themselves, staring at the floor, the ceiling, or out the window—anywhere except into the eyes of the people in the space they share. Why? Because they are trying to ignore, minimize, and refute the undesired, uncomfortable intimacy.

Have you ever traveled to another country? It's interesting that different cultures have different levels of comfort with personal space. For example, a recent study showed that in Argentina, people stand approximately 2.5 feet away when talking to strangers.[15] Compare that distance to the one in Romania, where people give strangers a much wider berth, typically standing 4.5 feet away. Throw COVID-19 into the mix, and the general advice—at least here in the United States—was to stand six feet apart from one another.

However, depending on the circumstances, such as being in an elevator with a stranger, even a six-foot separation can still feel intimate. Like all animals, we are designed to be on alert when other people are nearby, particularly strangers.

In this chapter, we are going to get up close and personal with physical intimacy. We'll explore the many ways it shows up in our daily lives and relationships, especially the way it affects our romantic relationships. Then I'll show you how you can experience physical intimacy in ways that are fun, flirty, and freeing.

---

[15] Melanie Radzicki McManus, "Which Countries Have the Smallest Personal Space?," HowStuffWorks Science (HowStuffWorks, March 25, 2022), https://science.howstuffworks.com/life/inside-the-mind/human-brain/which-countries-have-smallest-personal-space.htm.

Men, Women, and Proximity

If you're like most people, your default definition of physical intimacy probably involves touch. So I want to talk for a second about the times touch *isn't* involved.

Individuals vary greatly in their opinions of what constitutes physical intimacy without touch. Research has shown some interesting divides between men and women. According to sociologist Harry Brod, "Numerous studies have established that men are more likely to define emotional closeness as working or playing side by side, while women often view it as talking face to face."[16] Women also display more of what are called "general immediacy behaviors" during a conversation, such as leaning forward, nodding their head, smiling, and—wait for it—touching.

(I know I said we weren't going to talk about touch yet. Don't @ me![17])

However, these preferences can also work in the opposite direction, helping us understand what men and women *don't* like. Women are often more uncomfortable if a stranger sits next to them, whereas men tend to feel more discomfort if a stranger sits across from them.

There are different theories for why men and women prefer these different physical positions. It may be because, in general, women are more

> Women are often more uncomfortable if a stranger sits next to them, whereas men tend to feel more discomfort if a stranger sits across from them.

---

[16] Audrey Nelson PhD, "Why You Stand Side-by-Side or Face-to-Face," *Psychology Today* (Sussex Publishers, April 27, 2014), https://www.psychologytoday.com/us/blog/he-speaks-she-speaks/201404/why-you-stand-side-side-or-face-face.

[17] My editor added this. I guess it's what the kids say these days. I'm so stubborn, I didn't want to take it out just 'cause I'm old and had no idea what it was. For all you other old folks, "Don't @ me" is a playful way to say, "Don't come after me!" or "No offense!" Guess we learn something new every day!

worried about being physically attacked than men are, so when a man they don't know sits next to them, their inability to watch the stranger can put them on high alert. For men, direct eye contact may trigger some primal form of aggression—a throwback to a hunter staring down his prey.

Of course, these are not usually things you consciously think about when you're choosing your seat on the train. But I find it fascinating to reflect on the preferences and tendencies that are so deeply ingrained in us that we don't notice or question them.

Out of Sight but Still Physically Intimate

Okay, I know it's a bit weird to talk about bathroom habits, but I think it's the perfect real-life example of how physical intimacy can exist even when "privacy" is protected by doors and walls.[18] While women's restrooms generally offer individual cubicles, many women are still so uncomfortable with the physical proximity (intimacy) of others that they are hesitant to engage in the most normal of bodily functions, i.e., farting, peeing, and pooping. (I know men and women who do everything in their power to avoid using a public restroom because they find it almost unbearable!)

Heck, none of us are immune to this. In the airport the other day, I was having some—ahem—intestinal issues (so polite, right?). Even though I was in a stall with a door that closed completely—no gaps, thank goodness—I literally covered my face with my hands in embarrassment as my body made all sorts of gross noises that I couldn't pretend were going unnoticed. All I could think of was this book and how vulnerable I felt, despite the fact that no one could actually see me. I felt completely exposed and horribly mortified. In fact, I stayed

---

[18] Wow . . . did you ever imagine that a book about intimate relationships would include a discussion of bathroom habits? This is the way my mind works: nothing is ever taken for granted!

in the stall for several minutes after my body quieted down, hoping that anyone who had heard me would be long gone before I showed my face!

Again, just 'cause we're old doesn't mean we aren't silly. Or shy. And even though we won't get to emotional intimacy until the next chapter, let's just say that my sharing my bathroom travails with you is pretty emotionally intimate! (cringe)

In all seriousness, the bathroom examples are important because it's clear that there's nothing that is inherently comfortable or uncomfortable—no specific rule that can determine what is or isn't physical intimacy. It is highly subjective.

While this makes it hard for me to describe and define physical intimacy, it's actually great news for you. It presents a golden opportunity for you to get to know yourself more clearly. How do you define physical intimacy for yourself? What makes you comfortable or uncomfortable during a conversation? In what ways does that change when you're conversing with a family member versus a friend versus a stranger (or does it change at all)? How close is too close? When does proximity to someone make you feel warm and safe? When does it make your breath catch or your skin crawl?

If we have any hope of successfully explaining what we need or want or *don't* want, we have to learn to articulate what makes us uncomfortable. You're not "wrong" for feeling uneasy or unsettled by certain kinds of physical intimacy. You're human!

Plus, guess what? Your personal preferences, likes, and dislikes are going to surface in your romantic relationships too.

The Push-Pull of Physical Intimacy in Relationships

There are all sorts of fascinating contradictions within the realm of physical intimacy—or, at least, things we *perceive* to be contradictions.

A couple in the midst of a fight might climb into their shared bed (undeniable physical intimacy) and immediately turn their backs on

42

each other, effectively ignoring the intimacy inside their small shared space. A couple in the midst of a divorce might continue to share their house until one (or both of them) acquires the means to move out. This is uncomfortable, obviously, because while they are trying to end their relationship and cut their ties, they're still experiencing physical intimacy but trying to act like it's nothing.

When couples live together, they're actually fairly immersed in physical intimacy. Yet most fail to acknowledge or enjoy it. They have proximity, but paradoxically, it's not bringing them closer. They're basically just coexisting. It's like two people walking through a beautiful garden, so busy on their phones that they don't notice the beauty, the scents, the blooms, the butterflies. They waste a million opportunities to celebrate, marvel, and indulge with each other.

Here's the thing: most relationships, especially romantic ones, are almost always better off when you appreciate and *increase positive physical intimacy.*

The More You Touch, the Healthier You'll Be

We talked about this earlier, but it's worth repeating: Being physically affectionate with your partner doesn't just make you *feel* good, it's also good for your health. This isn't just loosey-goosey anecdotal optimism; it's science. Research proves that loving touches increase our levels of oxytocin, the hormone that stimulates our urge to bond. They also reduce cortisol, the stress hormone that increases our heart rate and blood pressure. And as if that weren't enough, physical affection decreases symptoms of physical problems, including back pain, muscle aches, insomnia, headaches, upset stomach, and even rashes and skin irritation.[19]

---

[19] "The Often-Overlooked Importance of Physical Intimacy," Family Institute, March 22, 2018, https://www.family-institute.org/behavioral-health-resources/magic-touch.

Failure to Thrive

I encourage my clients to add lots of deliberate, intentional physical touch *for the sole purpose of touching each other*. Not as a gateway to sex. Not as an obligation. For pure, unadulterated pleasure. I advocate for physical touch not because I'm expecting it to lead to something more but because I think you deserve the enormous pleasure it provides in and of itself. If you think I'm exaggerating, just ask anyone with a pet about the pleasure of nonsexual touch!

> Don't forget that physical intimacy is just as important as emotional or sexual intimacy in a relationship, even if that's not what most of us have been taught.

Don't forget that physical intimacy is just as important as emotional or sexual intimacy in a relationship, even if that's not what most of us have been taught.

I won't be surprised if this surprises you! After all, only a few generations ago, parents believed they were helping their kids by not touching or physically comforting them.[20] Physical affection was thought to weaken a child; independence was the method and the goal. But thanks to Dr. Harry Harlow's landmark studies with infant monkeys, the vital importance of maternal touch was confirmed. The world has finally recognized that physical connection is actually more important than food to a developing youngster.[21] Or, as the experts say today, lack of touch can cause a "failure to thrive."

---

[20] "Harlow's Classic Studies Revealed the Importance of Maternal Contact," Association for Psychological Science, June 20, 2018, https://www.psychologicalscience.org/publications/observer/obsonline/harlows-classic-studies-revealed-the-importance-of-maternal-contact.html.

[21] H.F. Harlow, R.O. Dodsworth, and M.K. Harlow, "Total Social Isolation in Monkeys," Proceedings of the National Academy of Sciences of the United States of America (U.S. National Library of Medicine, July 1965), https://www.ncbi.nlm.nih.gov/pmc/articles/PMC285801/.

Personally, I wish Dr. Harlow had pursued a few additional studies on the lack of physical intimacy in adults. While scientific research is still ongoing, anecdotal experience has already proved again and again that separation, such as physical distance or living apart for a long period of time, can be devastating. A loss of this kind of intimacy may easily dismantle a romantic relationship, no matter how much you love your partner.

Don't Stop Just Because It Feels Good

It's usually after I explain this to couples that I'll hear the most common excuse for resistance: "If we hug or just touch each other, I get turned on. I can't help it. Plus, it's frustrating to want them when they don't want me. So I'd rather not touch them at all until they're interested in getting sexy."

Hey, I get it.

But I reply, "Wow. Isn't it cool that you're wanted so much that even a simple touch gets a standing ovation?" (wink, wink)

Trying to avoid sexual arousal isn't a good reason to avoid touching each other. In fact, the opposite might be true. It could be healthy for the sexually enthusiastic partner to practice lots of physical intimacy so that their heart and body acclimate to the pleasure of nonsexual touches.

By the way, if you believe this is just a problem for "overly horny people," you're wrong. If this is something you struggle with, don't think you're alone or that it speaks poorly of you. There should be no shame in having a bodily reaction. Penile erections are no different than nipple erections, and we all know how welcome the latter are, even on mainstream TV.

While I certainly can't speak for anyone except myself, I will tell you that because I didn't grow up experiencing or witnessing familial physical affection other than that for infants, I thought touch belonged within the confines of a romantic or sexual relationship. In all honesty,

I spent decades giving awkward hugs to my friends—and avoiding them altogether with people I didn't know well. It sounds crazy, but it's true: I thought all touch was sexual.

Maybe it's TMI, but I even told a counselor that I could never be comfortable hugging a woman because how was I supposed to ignore the fact that our boobs would be squished together?[22] Yeah, we are all our own special kind of crazy, right? Thank goodness we can grow up to be whatever we choose!

I'd also be remiss if I didn't mention that associating physical touch with sex is a common response for those who have experienced sexual trauma. It takes a huge amount of fortitude and gumption to retrain yourself when history has taught you that safety isn't guaranteed.

I want to be clear: I'm not advocating your learning to appreciate physical intimacy for any reason other than the fact that you deserve the joyful comfort and connection that you, as a human, were programmed to desire. Remember, you're *wired* to reap the benefits of touch: the happy, lovey-dovey hormones and the alleviation of stress.

Now that you're on board with the importance of physical intimacy to you individually as well as to your relationship, let's think about how you can incorporate more of it into your life.

The Way We Touch

We all have different preferences when it comes to expressions of physical intimacy with the people we love.

You might be someone who is very comfortable with physical intimacy. You might enjoy being as physically close to your partner as possible and touching every chance you get. If so, you probably adore

---

[22] I have to share my editor's response to me when she read this for the first time: "P.S. If we ever hug (and I hope we do!), you will not have to worry about this because my boobs are really too small for squishing." This is the kind of support you can find when you are willing to allow intimacy into your life.

holding hands, giving back rubs, and resting your head quietly on their shoulder.

Even in non-romantic relationships, you might (or might not) enjoy sitting side by side with a close friend as you watch movies and share popcorn. You may find yourself being more productive if you're in physical proximity to others at work or at home: sitting in the same room with a coworker who's typing, or in your living room with your kid who's doing homework or (more likely) tapping away at their phone.

Or you might be someone who is less comfortable with touching. You might find physical affection requires a lot of deliberate effort. Some of my clients have told me that acts such as holding hands and snuggling make them feel vulnerable, clingy, and/or needy, so they avoid them like the plague.

Your comfort with and desire for touch probably has something to do with the way you grew up—but your family of origin doesn't have to dictate your preferences forever.

For example, I grew up in a family that was extremely touch avoidant. My parents rarely hugged me or my siblings, and we siblings never touched each other unless we were fighting. This behavior was true for my extended family as well (where do you think my parents learned it?). My grandmothers hugged us hello and goodbye, and even those exchanges were *incredibly awkward!*

In elementary school, I read a book about a mom dying suddenly, so I decided I was going to start kissing my mom good night each evening, even though it felt weird for both of us. As she sat in her favorite reading chair, I'd lean over the arm and give her cheek a quick peck. It was so discombobulating for both of us that we never acknowledged it. I stopped doing it sometime in high school.

Those of you who grew up being cuddled and snuggled probably find this level of ineptitude ridiculous, but sadly, it's not as uncommon as I wish it were.

It shouldn't surprise you that this lack of affection left me starved for touch. But as much as I craved it, I was still very awkward when it came to physical intimacy outside a romantic relationship. When I was in college, I literally had to teach myself to hug my friends!

I tell you this because I want you to know that just because intimacy doesn't come easily to us, it doesn't mean we don't want it. Better yet, it doesn't mean we can't learn to excel in it, even as we are continuously trying to improve.

Everyone, including you, can learn to enjoy each kind of intimacy. All it takes is a willingness to stretch yourself, a refusal to let awkwardness stop you, and a commitment to ongoing practice.

That being said, it's to be expected that individuals are going to vary widely in what and how much satisfies their need for each kind of intimacy. This doesn't have to be a problem, but it can become one when the relationship defaults or "settles" for the lowest common denominator—that is, when the one who desires the *least* amount controls it.

> Everyone, including you, can learn to enjoy each kind of intimacy. All it takes is a willingness to stretch yourself, a refusal to let awkwardness stop you, and a commitment to ongoing practice.

Think of this in terms of TV volume. Let's say Davon has great hearing, so she likes the volume at level four, but Kade's hearing isn't that good anymore, so he wants it turned up to eight. Since in this scenario the lowest level wins, Kade can't hear the whole show. He's left frustrated, and his level of frustration builds day by day until it becomes serious resentment. Meanwhile, Davon is confused because she thinks the volume is fine; she doesn't understand why Kade doesn't just relax and enjoy the show!

Here's how this might show up in regard to physical intimacy: Shawn craves morning snuggles before getting out of bed because they cause him to go to work with a smile, but his partner, Kendal, starts worrying about her to-do list as soon as the alarm goes off, so she finds morning snuggles annoying. You're probably not surprised to learn that annoyance avoidance beats desire, so morning snuggles don't happen. Kendal starts tackling her list like a pro, but poor Shawn goes to work every day feeling rejected. Can you guess what happens at night when Kendal is ready for a celebratory hug before dinner?

I'd never suggest that there is a specific amount of physical intimacy you and your partner should have. The point is that every relationship needs its own special sauce, and those involved are the only ones who can create it. It takes a lot of attention to detail because each partner has to know themself well enough to be honest about their needs. Then they have to work together to find a creative way to satisfy both partners without depleting either.

They Call It *Natural* for a Reason

Let's imagine that you and yours have found your way to your favorite beach where you're holding hands as you meander along the shoreline, enjoying some warm hugs, a few delightful kisses, and some soulful eye gazing.

Your heart is happy—and then you notice that it's not just his heart that's happy . . . Will you forgive me for saying there are no hard rules? (Couldn't help myself, ha-ha-ha!)

Some therapists will say, "When you hug or kiss your partner outside of sexual activity, try not to become aroused."

To that I reply, *no way!* If you're aroused, that's okay! Yes, I want kissing and physical closeness to be appreciated on its own and not to carry any obligation, especially if you agreed beforehand that it wasn't going to lead to sexy stuff. But I refuse to buy into the idea that one person's arousal creates another person's obligation. There is no reason erotic arousal should be a less valid sign of appreciation than a sigh of pleasure or a blissful melting into an embrace. Why should a natural arousal response deny a loving couple the pleasure of physical intimacy?

After all, it would take effort and energy to negate sexual arousal. They don't call it *natural* for nothin'! In other words, he'd have to deliberately avoid noticing the feel of her skin, the sensation of her body pressing against him, the scent of her shampoo. He'd have to disassociate from his physical experience. I'm trying to get you to do the exact opposite! I want both of you to milk every drop of pleasure you can from each delightful touch.

Why on earth would anyone suggest you pull back instead of lean in? The whole point is to connect!

I can't imagine saying, "Okay, hug your partner, but don't fully enjoy it." Enjoy it fully! Enjoy *your* pleasure. Enjoy *their* pleasure. Rejoice in the fact that your bodies enjoy each other so much. There's nothing negative about that.

That said, you'll want to make sure your desire doesn't create an obligation for your partner. But that's as simple as saying, "I want you to know that when I touch you, it's such a turn on. But I'm not demanding or even asking for sex. I just need you to know that to me, you are smokin' hot."

It's nice to be wanted. It's nice when we're able to see somebody's pleasure, to feel them melt into our arms. It feels so good. We feel so powerful. We're thrilled to be that important.

We have to get rid of the sense of shame people have around sexual arousal. That's just foolish. It is instinctual. It is natural. It is wonderful. So embrace it. Plus, once you both are skilled in each of the intimacies, you'll have lots of opportunities to blend physical and sexual intimacy!

Hey Body, How Are You?

Some of us talk to ourselves on a regular basis but ignore when our body tries to chime in.

Pause for a moment: What is your body saying? Can you "hear" anything?

If you close your eyes, take a deep breath, and still can't hear anything, it may be because you're not really listening. I don't say that to make you feel bad or ashamed. Most of us don't know how to listen to our bodies because we've been taught to ignore or override them. You know what I mean—it starts with parents telling us, "Oh, that doesn't really hurt that much," or that it's bad to touch ourselves in certain ways even though it feels good, teachers telling us it doesn't matter how long it takes to complete our homework it has to be done, bosses rolling their eyes when we beg for a few minutes to stretch our legs or grab lunch. There's no way to know whether your body got quiet or you just stopped listening, but one way or another, it's time to change things.

You don't need a partner to start tuning in to your body. Just give yourself a few minutes alone in a quiet place with your eyes closed. Allow your mind to focus on your legs, noticing if they're tense or relaxed. If you stretch them, what parts feel good? Is there any pain or discomfort? Does the movement give you the urge to repeat it or to move differently? Put your hands on your legs and note whether they're warm or cool before squeezing them. Allow yourself to decide if it's pleasurable or not, both from the perspective of your hands and your legs. Spend the time to get acquainted with all the other parts of your body, especially your erogenous zones, listening from the inside as well as stimulating from the outside. With practice, I think you'll find enormous comfort in being more attuned to your body. I know it will benefit from your attention and care.

As you focus on physical intimacy, even by yourself, feel free to notice and appreciate any erotic arousal, but don't let it shut you down. It can exist without requiring you to be distracted by it. Focus on all the sensory pleasures of touch rather than interpreting them as a means to an orgasmic end.

Start Intentionally Touching Each Other

If you're already enjoying lots of deliberate physical intimacy in your relationship—yay! Keep it up and see if you can get even more goodness from your proximity and touches by adding eye contact, whispered terms of endearment, or taking deep breaths together.

If you haven't been enjoying much physical intimacy together, start by committing to spending at least a minute a day touching in a way that feels good to both of you. Gradually increase the time and frequency of these deliberate touches. Also, notice those times when you're in close proximity to each other and suggest ways that you can bridge the gap together. Perhaps that's sliding your chairs closer together at meals, eating together on a banquette, or resting your legs on each other while sprawled on the couch.

One activity many couples rush to in the hope of developing more physical intimacy is massage. For some people, this can be a wonderful, rewarding way to connect. But it is not for everyone! Lots of people consider massage a sexual act, and since the goal is to focus on physical intimacy for its own sake, it might not be the best way to practice.

If you do decide to use massage, I suggest you focus on the physicality of it by asking yourself questions such as the following: What does it feel like to touch my partner's skin? How does it feel to relieve their tension? Am I relaxing into the massage as the tension is working its way out of my body?

It's also worth noting that for some people, massage can cause negative triggers, including body insecurity and shame. If a person is self-conscious about their body, then the deliberate exposure and touch of a massage might make them feel even more awkward or uncomfortable. Please make sure to discuss this with your partner instead of just assuming they're as into it as you are.

We all have our own likes and dislikes as well as our own baggage and triggers. Don't assume that your partner's comfort level with certain kinds of physical intimacy is the same as yours!

Touch as a (Not So) Secret Weapon

You can have all the intimacy possible with your partner, but you're still going to have disagreements, maybe even fights. These won't doom your relationship if you learn to handle them respectfully.

> It's really hard to fight with someone when you're holding hands.

While there are lots of other books specifically focused on how to "fight fair," I can't help but give you this one very simple yet effective suggestion: it's really hard to fight with someone when you're holding hands.

Go ahead; try it. My guess is that at the first sign of irritation, your partner will try to pull away. That's how you'll know I'm right!

Keep in mind that this doesn't mean you should ignore the rules of consent and force them to endure your touch. If they pull away, your best bet is to give them a moment to calm down before calmly expressing your desire to maintain a physical connection while you work through the emotional aspects of the issue. That might sound something like this: "I know you're upset, and I get it. I want us to deal with it even though it's difficult. Most of all, I want us both to remember that even though we disagree right now, we're on the same team. That's why I want to hold your hand as we talk this through. I don't want our anger to overshadow how much we love each other."

If they're too upset to touch while talking, you might consider taking a break until they are ready. In my experience, it's rare for couples to be as hurtful to each other while holding hands as they can be from across the room.

...Physical Intimacy Is Physically Impossible

Military spouses have been dealing with this issue forever, but these days, they aren't the only ones. While I'd like to assure you that the old adage "Absence makes the heart grow fonder" is true, reality indicates that it's probably only applicable to short-term separations. Long-term long-distance relationships are much harder to maintain than love songs would like us to believe.

However, this doesn't mean all long-distance relationships are doomed. It does mean that they require special "work-arounds," particularly with respect to physical intimacy. One often overlooked approach that has proved helpful to my clients is to engage their olfactory sense. Yep, that's a fancy way of saying that smelling your partner is a good way to help maintain your relationship if you can't touch each other.

I know this sounds weird, but it's true. Not only am I completely serious, but also, what I'm suggesting is backed by science.

Did you know that of all your senses, smell is the strongest memory trigger? Scents travel from your olfactory bulb directly to the amygdala and hippocampus in your brain.[23] These are the regions related to emotion and memory. That's why the smell of oatmeal cookies might immediately make you feel like you're back in your grandmother's kitchen or why a whiff of a particular men's cologne might immediately fill you with rage as you remember your ex who cheated on you.

Exchanging personally scented items with your partner is an easy, effective way to keep each of you in the other's mind and heart. Combining this with physical sensations can go a long way toward maintaining a close connection despite the distance. For example, you could give your partner a large stuffed animal wearing one of your

---

[23] Colleen Walsh, "What the Nose Knows," (Harvard Gazette, February 27, 2020), https://news.harvard.edu/gazette/story/2020/02/how-scent-emotion-and-memory-are-intertwined-and-exploited/.

well-worn shirts spritzed with your signature cologne. Daily hugs would give them "hits" of you that would keep you front of mind. An alternative is giving them a blanket you've slept with so they'll smell you all night long. (Even better, make it a personalized blanket with your picture on it like one of my clients did!)

There are a number of creative ways to fulfill the need for touch without risking your relationship. One possibility would be for you and your partner to create a list of approved "suitable substitutions": others who can provide fulfilling physical intimacy without violating the parameters of your relationship. They could include nearby pets, kids appointed as "official huggers," platonic friends who will serve as your snuggle buddy during movies or lonely nights at home, professional massage therapists, elderly neighbors who may also be touch deprived. The list is endless. (Note that it's also important to specify exactly what kinds of touch are acceptable and from whom.)

If you are committed and willing to be creative, there are lots of options to overcome the miles. Although none of the other intimacies can be substituted, an abundance in other areas will help carry you through this lapse. With that in mind, even though you may not be able to do the exercises at the end of this book exactly as written, feel free to adapt them to your particular situation.

Moving onward, let's look at the more enigmatic side of intimacy. Now's your chance to let your emotions run free!

Tantalizing Takeaways

- Note—physical intimacy isn't just about sex!
- Affectionate touches improve your emotional and physical health
- Above all, remember that most relationships, especially romantic ones, benefit when you *increase positive physical intimacy.*

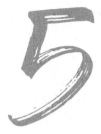

Your Emotional Side
Is Magnetic

When we reveal our—or witness someone else's—emotional vulnerability, their deep-seated feelings, fears, hopes, dreams, or dread, **emotional intimacy** is created. In these moments, one's inner self is seen or exposed, regardless of whether or not it's acknowledged. This can occur via conversation, tears, emotional outbursts, or other vulnerable expressions of self—even when we aren't seeking intimacy. In this chapter, we'll dig into some of the common roadblocks that people struggle with and ways to choose to be emotionally intimate as a path to a deeper connection.

***

Hey, wait! Don't put the book down now!

I know we're diving into murky waters here by focusing on emotions, which might be really, really uncomfortable for you. However, I hope you'll trust me enough to give me a chance to make things easier for you, even if you're fighting a strong urge to chuck this book across the room or conveniently "lose" it—or, more likely, to skip this chapter on your race to get to the sexy stuff!

You'd be surprised to learn how many people get stressed out when I start talking about emotional intimacy. It's a bit like the reaction to Voldemort's name in the Harry Potter books: We pretend that refusing to acknowledge it makes it less real. Ha!

The good news is, if you'll stick with me, I think I can help you to easily get over your emotion phobia.

Whew! I'm glad you're still here. You rock!

Okay, now that we both know that you can do this, let's change your life.

Quick "Test" for Emotional Intimacy

If you're wondering how to determine whether or not you have emotional intimacy in your relationship, ask yourself this: When something happens that makes me feel really good or really bad, does sharing it with my partner make me feel better?

To clarify, this isn't a question of whether or not your partner solves problems for you. It's about determining if the mere act of sharing your feelings with them is uplifting.

If your answer is a resounding *yes,* then you probably have a healthy level of emotional intimacy, which will become even deeper as you make your way through this book.

If your answer is "usually," then you're on the right track; just keep reading!

Any other response is probably an indication that you'll benefit significantly from focusing on this chapter.

When Silence Is Safety

When I say, "Let's change your life," it might sound like I'm exaggerating. I'm really not.

What you're about to learn about emotional intimacy won't transform just your romantic relationships; it can transform *all* your relationships.

You'll see opportunities to create emotional intimacy, and you may well recognize how emotional intimacy, or a lack thereof, affected situations in your past.

Are you racking your brain trying to figure out what I mean by "emotional intimacy"? If so, you're not the only one. Most people are a bit uncertain but let me try to make it easier. In casual terms, emotional intimacy is when someone has insight (intentional or not) into parts of your psyche that you consider personal or private. Or, you into theirs. Once emotional intimacy is established, its effect is dependent on the behavior of those involved.

> Men often feel emotional intimacy when they are allowed to simply exist in somebody else's physical presence without having to make conversation, respond to conversation, or prove themselves in any way.

We use emotional intimacy in any number of ways, such as simply calling our spouse to check in after a big meeting they had been worried about. Or, taking one look at our partner's face when they walk in the door and immediately telling the kids to leave them alone for a few minutes because they've had a hard day.

The longer your relationship, the more emotional intimacy you're likely to share, even if you don't put it to good use. My hope is that regardless of your current situation, you will focus on creating even more emotional intimacy together and use it to foster a stronger sense of connection.

While many women feel comfortable creating emotional intimacy through talking, crying, sharing, or laughing together, men often feel emotional intimacy when they are allowed to simply exist in somebody else's physical presence without having to make conversation, respond to conversation, or prove themselves in any way. This sounds bizarre to women because we tend to think that if someone isn't talking to us, it's because they'd rather be alone.

But that's not the way men generally operate. They've grown up being told that what they do determines their worth, which is exhausting. It means that when they are around others, they are constantly trying to *accomplish* something. When they are with someone they don't feel compelled to impress, they are finally able to relax. They can let their guard down and simply be themselves. To be loved without doing— that's emotionally intimate to more men than I can count.[24]

By way of example, Nora and Byron often had breakfast together. During breakfast, Byron liked to read the news quietly. Nora found the silence uncomfortable, so she regularly tried to make conversation. Byron typically responded distractedly and quickly returned to his newspaper. This seriously irritated Nora; she resented the idea that Byron was more interested in the news than he was in her. As soon as she finished eating, she would leave the table. Only then would Byron say, "Oh, no, please don't go. Stay with me; I like having you here."

This drove Nora nuts! She felt Byron was being disrespectful to her, expecting her to sit around waiting until he wanted something. Clearly, if he valued her company, he'd engage with her. He was always the life of the party with their friends, so it seemed obvious to her that he was more interested in them than her these days.

When Nora and Byron heard me talk about emotional intimacy, the light bulb went on for both of them: Byron felt emotionally intimate when Nora allowed him to be present but quiet!

From that day on, Nora understood that she was Byron's safe harbor. He felt safe enough with her to be with her without having to impress her. In those times, he felt emotionally intimate because he felt wholly accepted. He didn't need conversation to establish emotional intimacy. He needed the comfort of not having to prove himself. He

---

[24] Note that I am speaking generally about the differences between genders, not universally. There will be any number of individuals to whom these generalities don't apply.

needed to be loved for being himself, which felt pretty perfect to him. As for Nora, learning that her presence allowed Byron to relax gave her a special sense of pride and joy. Interestingly, she likened it to the pleasure she felt when her children wanted her to tuck them in rather than anyone else.

Oh, This Is Awkward . . .

Like the forced physical intimacy that occurs in a crowded elevator, emotional intimacy is not always invited, intentional, or wanted.

Have you ever stumbled upon an acquaintance or stranger crying, talking to themselves, or sneaking a cigarette? Despite the fact that you didn't do anything wrong, you may have found yourself feeling uncomfortable and looking away. That's how emotional intimacy sneaks into our life, even if we try to avoid it.

It doesn't matter if the other person knows you saw them; intimacy doesn't have to be mutual to exist. In fact, many experiences of emotional intimacy take place when we chance upon someone's secret or private moment. Even if they're brief, even if we wish they didn't happen, even if we try to forget about them, they're real. As much as we might wish we could "unsee" them, we're stuck. Annoyingly, the more intense our reaction, the more lasting the memory. (How many adults still cringe when thinking about the time they caught their parents "doing it"?!)

As for looking away? Well, that's a very typical reaction for all of us. Except for children.

We aren't born with a disdain for intimacy. It's the opposite. As we talked about earlier, humans are wired to seek intimate connections. Only as we age are we taught to fight those natural instincts. Personally, I love it when children force their parents to acknowledge emotional intimacy by asking things like, "Why is that man crying?" We'd all be a lot happier if we learned how to face these situations with kindness and curiosity, asking the crying man, "How can I help you?" instead of shushing our child while scurrying away.

What's so telling about the power of intimacy is that we literally have to look away from it to distance ourselves from it.

I'll never forget a flight I was on years ago. Just after landing, a young woman received a phone call notifying her of a relative's death. She began sobbing as she asked the caller what had happened, trying to make sense of the unexpected news. In a matter of minutes, everyone around her had stopped talking. We all began fidgeting uncomfortably, looking everywhere but at her. Soon, the entire plane was enveloped in total silence. The tension was palpable.

As she continued weeping, the rest of us quietly gathered our belongings before slowly deplaning. Other than her sobs and a few simple condolences, "I'm sorry for your loss," the plane was silent. This woman's grief was so powerful that we were all consumed with sorrow. None of us wanted this unexpected emotional intimacy, yet we couldn't avoid it. Nor did we know how to deal with it.

Looking back, I hate that I didn't make my way over to her so I could hold her while she cried. I know she needed that. But I told myself she wouldn't want to cry on a stranger's shoulder. In hindsight, that says more about my level of comfort with emotional intimacy than hers since I didn't even make the offer.

You've probably experienced something similar in your life but didn't know how to explain it. Now that you're learning about emotional intimacy, I expect you'll suddenly have clarity about any number of situations in your past, not to mention your future.

> The power of emotional intimacy is that we literally have to look away from it to distance ourselves from it. The moment may be fleeting but it causes intense feelings that can stay for a long time.

That's the power of emotional intimacy. The moment itself may be fleeting, but it causes intense feelings that can stay with you for a very long time.

Caution: Highly Flammable!

Emotional intimacy can sometimes feel like walking through a minefield, especially if you've been betrayed by those you've trusted, had your heart broken by someone you loved, or simply been let go by people you valued.

> Heartbreak sucks, but it doesn't have to be permanent. Your heart can heal, just like your arm or leg.

The truth is, we've all been hurt, and not just in romantic relationships; we've *also* been disappointed by friends or let down by our parents. Even those with the best intentions can hurt our feelings or break our hearts.

When those things happen, especially time after time, it's perfectly rational for your brain to find ways to avoid experiencing this pain again in the future. It can seem reasonable to conclude that avoiding emotional intimacy will keep you safe.

But here's what I want you to remind your brain:

Heartbreak sucks, but it doesn't have to be permanent. Your heart can heal, just like your arm or leg.

Have you ever known anyone who has run a marathon? It's not uncommon for a marathoner to invest a lot of effort in planning the best training schedule, as well as diet, before spending months practicing, only to be sidelined for some period of time due to a painful injury. They'll tell you it's practically a miracle if they actually cross the finish line (even if it's not the first marathon they trained for) because their body has been through the wringer. But they'll also tell you that they'd happily do it all over again. Despite everything they went through, it was worth it.

Loving relationships are no different.

Sure, some people make their first significant romantic relationship work for a lifetime, but it takes most of us a few tries before we find a race and pace that works for us.

Clearly, running isn't for everyone; some of us (like me!) are perfectly happy standing on the sidelines. But human nature is such that very few of us are truly happy being sidelined when it comes to love.

Throughout three decades of working with individuals and couples, I've met thousands of people who were eager to tell me all the good reasons they had for giving up on intimate relationships, romantic and otherwise. Among the most popular are these:

- I don't need anyone else to be happy.
- All the good ones are taken.
- Everyone is just looking for sex (or a free meal).
- They're all cheaters and can't be trusted.
- I'm too _____ (old, heavy, picky, set in my ways, etc.).
- It's too much work.
- I've tried everything; it's hopeless.

I always listen. I tell them I understand. But what I understand is probably different than what they're thinking.

I know that most of those reasons are code for "I'd rather give up hope of having a happy, healthy relationship than risk failing, being disappointed, or getting hurt. I also don't want to admit that I'm afraid of those things, so I'm just going to pretend I don't want love."

Sometimes if I meet someone I think might be open to a little inspiration, I tell them about my friend Laura, who really wanted to run a marathon. For years, every time Laura would get geared up for one, something would happen to derail her. She was beyond frustrated; she told everyone she was cursed. But, by George, if she didn't keep trying!

A full decade after her first failed effort, she finally did it. You would have thought she'd just won the Olympic gold medal when she crossed the finish line! Twenty years later, she's run several more marathons despite the huge toll they take on her body. Laura says she was born to run; she's got so much moxie that she thinks the obstacles are there to make sure she never takes it for granted!

If you've been standing on the sidelines, avoiding relationships or intimacy, I hope you'll be inspired by Laura. Give yourself grace to persevere through the struggles, and remind yourself that you, like all the rest of us, were born for intimate relationships. Even though it takes a lot of hard work and painful injuries may sideline you for a bit, your efforts will pay off sooner or later. When they do, the rewards will make it all worthwhile.

Running a Three-Legged Marathon

When I give talks about intimacy, I notice lots of married couples nodding along, exchanging proud looks with their partner. They're pleased that they're clearly "in the race" by virtue of their relationship status.

Unfortunately, I can see their expressions quickly change when I ask them to share any recent experiences involving emotional intimacy with their spouse. Suddenly they realize that simply being partnered doesn't mean they are succeeding at intimacy.

What's really sad is that it's often the formalizing of a relationship (moving in together or marrying) that instigates the decline of fulfilling intimacy for couples.

Remember what Laura said about obstacles making her appreciate running marathons? When it comes to your relationship, do you see the obstacles as signs to work harder and smarter? Or do you take them as signs that you should quit?[25]

In every relationship, no matter how wonderful it is, you have a choice: You can rely on the NRE (new relationship energy) that brought

---

[25] I'm certainly not suggesting anyone should ignore serious red flags! Only that not all issues are inherently dangerous or unimprovable.

you together, hoping it's enough to get you across the finish line decades later. Or you can commit to a training routine designed to strengthen the intimacy needed to keep your love alive.

If you choose the latter, you'll have to learn not only what *you* want, need, and desire but also what works for your partner.

Yep, there's the rub. While running a marathon is just about *you,* you're only half of your relationship. This means, just as Gary Chapman showed us in *The 5 Love Languages,* it's likely that your partner will have their own unique needs that must be attended to for you both to "finish the race" together.

In other words, creating a lovingly intimate relationship is probably even harder than running a marathon. It's more like running a *three-legged* marathon! If you don't lean in, work together, and support each other, it's not going to work.

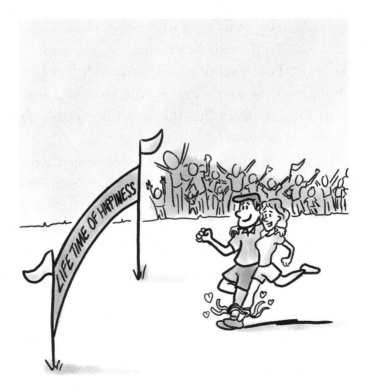

The reward, though, can be a lifetime of happiness, which is better than any marathon prize I've ever heard of. Plus, being a marathon runner can be lonely. The advantage of being partnered is that your pleasures are magnified because they're shared. And what's more, your struggles are lessened by sharing. When you think of your relationship as a three-legged marathon, it becomes clear that success—your happiness—requires moving *toward* your partner rather than pulling away.

> When you think of your relationship as a three-legged marathon, it becomes clear that success—your happiness—requires moving *toward* your partner rather than pulling away.

Basketball's Dynamic Duo

Almost weekly, I hear, "How am I supposed to know what they want? I'm not a mind reader!" My response is always, "You're not supposed to be a mind reader; you're supposed to have enough emotional intimacy to make an educated guess." When men look at me in confusion, I offer the example of Magic Johnson and Kareem Abdul-Jabbar. This dynamic duo won five championships together while playing for the Los Angeles Lakers and they are regarded as one of the most successful pairings in basketball history. Although, frankly, you can look at the relationships between members of any winning basketball or soccer team.

Athletic teams don't talk about emotional intimacy, but they rely on it nevertheless.

Watch any great team, and you'll notice that each member is fully aware of what their teammates are doing at any given time. You'll see them pass the ball to one another with barely a glance. Their confidence comes from an almost innate sense of where their teammates will be. This is based on *knowing* one another, which is just a casual way of describing emotional intimacy. They also use emotional intimacy to anticipate their opponent's actions. They learn what intimidation tactics are the most effective, how they are likely to respond to different challenges, etc. There's no way to do this other than to delve into a person's psyche.

In short, when it comes to almost any competition, natural talent is helpful, but being skilled in emotional intimacy is what makes a champion. This is true in sports, life, and love.

That, in a nutshell, is what emotional intimacy is all about. Get to know your partner. Study them closely—not just what they willingly share but also what they don't. You may even be able to discover what they don't yet understand about themself.

Heck, maybe emotional intimacy will make you a mind reader after all!

The Odds Are Against You

This section gets a TW (trigger warning)! Gender stereotypes to follow.

Again, please don't cancel me! I'm not suggesting these stereotypes are healthy or should be continued. I'm simply recognizing that they exist. Our only hope of changing things is to acknowledge them so we can tackle 'em directly.

That being said, most heterosexual romantic relationships are set up for failure.

Sounds harsh, I know. Especially because I'm such an optimistic romantic. But it's the truth.

Let me explain the problem:

Men are generally taught to avoid *emotional* intimacy unless or until they are in the midst of *sexual* intimacy. Then they can be mushy, gushy ("I love you," "I love the way you feel," "I

> Men are generally taught to avoid *emotional* intimacy unless or until they are in the midst of *sexual* intimacy. Then they can be mushy, gushy ("I love you," "I love the way you feel," "I never want to leave you").

never want to leave you"). Heck, even the king of England confessed he wanted to be a tampon inside the woman he loved![26]

And in case you've forgotten (or never heard of) Tampongate, here's the transcript of the secret phone call that scandalized the British royal family and the rest of the world in 1993:

CHARLES: Oh stop! I want to feel my way along you, all over you and up and down you and in and out . . .
CAMILLA: Oh!
CHARLES: Particularly in and out.
CAMILLA: Oh, that's just what I need at the moment.
CHARLES: Is it?
CHARLES: Oh, God. I'll just live inside your trousers or something. It would be much easier!
CAMILLA: (laughing) What are you going to turn into, a pair of knickers? (Both laugh). Oh, you're going to come back as a pair of knickers.
CHARLES: Or, God forbid, a Tampax. Just my luck! (Laughs)
CAMILLA: You are a complete idiot! (Laughs) Oh, what a wonderful idea.

I share this with appreciation for the emotionally expressive King of England. I applaud his desire (awkward though it may be) to love and be intimate with his beloved. I'm not laughing at him—I'm laughing *with* him. And while I don't condone cheating, I do appreciate love and longing.

Women, on the other hand, are generally taught to avoid *sexual* intimacy unless or until they have *emotional* intimacy. Even then, we are taught to use sexual intimacy as a reward for our partner rather than for our own pleasure.

---

[26] Personally, I despise the invasion of privacy that led to this disclosure, but I applaud Charles for being so emotionally attuned and expressive. It's a horrible waste that despite his feelings for Camilla, he didn't find a way to marry her before Diana became collateral damage. https://www.thecut.com/2020/05/no-tampongate-in-the-crown-josh-oconnor.html.

Maybe that statement offends you. Maybe you think I'm a bad feminist for mentioning it. After all, it's bold and it's ugly, but—in my experience—it's absolutely true. And important.

This is why so much of my coaching work is spent teaching men how to enjoy more intimacy with their clothes on and women to enjoy more intimacy with their clothes off. Both are key. Both are equally important.

It's like the age-old chicken versus the egg question: it's not obvious which one comes first. (Let's just ignore that pun, shall we?)

In all seriousness, many people, including a lot of relationship experts, think it's okay to ignore a lack of sexual intimacy in a marriage while they focus on the emotional aspects of the relationship. But I think that's just as harmful as tolerating a lack of emotional intimacy while improving the sexual aspects.

Let me put it this way: What advice would you give a woman who is distraught because her husband has refused to talk with her for three weeks despite her efforts to engage him in conversation? Would your advice be the same to a man who is distraught because his wife has refused to engage in sexual intimacy for the past three weeks despite his requests?

> Women are generally taught to avoid *sexual* intimacy unless or until they have *emotional* intimacy. Even then, we are taught to use sexual intimacy as a reward for our partner rather than for our own pleasure.

These insights aren't only for straight couples. They can be extremely illuminating for gay and queer couples too. Do you think two men who have great sexual intimacy but struggle to connect to each other emotionally are going to last? What about two women who are great at talking to each other but aren't comfortable being naked together?

I think this is an important discussion to have because the bias is so widespread. It creates the expectation that emotional intimacy is imperative in a marriage, but sexual intimacy is optional. In most hetero relationships particularly, it's seen as perfectly reasonable for a wife to feel entitled to emotional intimacy throughout every phase of a marriage, even if she wants it daily. Yet if her husband asks for sexual intimacy on a daily basis, she's likely to feel entitled to laugh in his face while telling him there's no way that's ever going to happen. She might even go further, calling him self-centered for wanting that from her when she's already got so many other things to take care of, such as her job, their kids, the house. In her mind, his desire for sexual intimacy is selfish. She thinks of sex as an optional form of entertainment or a means to an orgasm—for *him*. She doesn't recognize sexual intimacy as a vital part of their relationship, something that benefits her as well as her husband. She doesn't realize it can be a mutually joyful way to solidify and improve their alliance. She is completely blind to the fact that sexual intimacy is as valid a form of loving expression as a hug.

We have to acknowledge our cultural bias in favor of emotional intimacy in marriage. That bias can lead us to think that emotional intimacy is obvious and easy and that if we aren't getting enough of it, it's our partner's fault.

Please don't misunderstand me. It's totally cool for couples to prioritize different things in their relationship. But to do so, they should give full value to what matters to each of them, not minimize one arbitrarily.

The reason this is important for you to understand now is that, as we delve into the intricacies of emotional intimacy, we have to acknowledge our cultural bias in favor of emotional intimacy in marriage. That bias can lead us to think that emotional intimacy is obvious and easy and that if we aren't getting enough of it, it's our partner's fault.

Unfortunately, it's *not* that easy.

"I'd Like Some Emotional Intimacy, Please"

I'd be lying if I said I hear those six words from new clients. Here are some things I do hear:

- We never actually talk anymore.
- She doesn't want me like I want her.
- We aren't as close as we used to be.
- I feel like I don't even know them anymore.
- It's like we're living separate lives.
- I don't know if I love her anymore.
- He won't listen.
- She's so focused on the kids, it's like I don't exist other than to pay the bills.
- He doesn't understand me at all.
- I don't matter to her.
- I wish he'd try to comfort me when I've been having a rough time.

This list could go on for pages, but each line is an indication of the same problem: a lack of emotional intimacy in the relationship.

It wouldn't take an expert to suggest that if the complaint was truly as simple as a lack of conversation ("We don't talk"), you could fix it by spending ten minutes a day talking. But you and I both know that wouldn't fix anything.

Even once my clients understand that what they are craving is emotional intimacy, if they bring it up to their partner—especially if it's a man—the response is often along the lines of, "I don't even know what emotional intimacy is or what it would feel like. Just tell me what you want me to do, and I'll do it, dammit!"

I don't blame my clients for being offended by the aggressiveness of the response. But I also understand that it's annoying and scary when we are asked to do things we don't know how to do. It makes us feel "less than," so we're likely to project our feelings of insecurity onto the one putting us in the position of failing.

If a wife asks her husband for more emotional intimacy, he may feel like he's been thrown into a helicopter and told to fly it—when he's never even been in a chopper as a *passenger*, let alone a pilot. The poor guy might be willing to give it a shot—though I'd imagine his passengers would kindly request he not do so! But he has no idea where to begin. He doesn't have an instruction manual. He can't watch a YouTube video to learn the basics. He has no way of knowing if he is doing it the "right" way.

Make no mistake: I'm not saying emotional intimacy is something that women can master but that men can't. I'm not even saying women are better at it than men. All I'm saying is that we still live in a world that tends to encourage boys and men to ignore their emotions. They're expected to repress any desire to emotionally connect with others. Meanwhile, girls and women are allowed to be more comfortable and attuned to theirs. It's not surprising then that women tend to get a lot more practice with their emotions than men do.

You'd think that all this practice would make us really good at emotional intimacy, right? But you know what the most common response given to a husband's "Just tell me what you want me to do, and I'll do it" is?

"Ummmm . . . hmmmm . . . I guess, just ask about my day and listen when I tell you?"

Even if we're more fluent in the language of emotions than men are and more comfortable asking for emotional intimacy, we may not be great at either giving or getting it!

As a result, many heterosexual couples wind up in the aforementioned Catch-22: in relationships, men tend to seek sexual intimacy, believing that the emotional intimacy will follow, while most women seek emotional intimacy first and are only willing to entertain the idea of sexual intimacy once we feel emotionally fulfilled.

So how do we get on the same page? How do we deepen the emotional intimacy between us when we can't agree on how important it is or even what it looks and feels like?

Be More Childlike

First, let's set the record straight: All but a very few of us, regardless of our gender, are capable of emotional intimacy. Humans, with the possible exception of psychopaths or sociopaths, are created with the instinct and ability to form emotional bonds with others.

> All but a very few of us, regardless of our gender, are capable of emotional intimacy. Humans, with the possible exception of psychopaths or sociopaths, are created with the instinct and ability to form emotional bonds with others.

From the moment we're born, we instinctively seek emotional intimacy. Our survival depends on it. We need our parents to not just want a baby; we need them to want *us*. Given how difficult it is to take care of a newborn, it's understandable that nature cheats the system a bit by filling mothers with hormones that encourage them to bond with their babies until they, as children, are able to give more in return for the care they require. Wouldn't it be fantastic if we women got that chemical boost at our weddings too?

Hmm . . . wait a minute . . . didn't we just finish talking about how physical touch stimulates oxytocin? Isn't oxytocin the very same bonding hormone that helps keep new moms bonded to their crying babies? (Wow, maybe married couples should do drugs—oxytocin, that is!) I'm pretty sure this means that when your relationship is tough, you need more touch.

Of course, touch won't make up for a lack of emotional intimacy, but just like parental bonds begin with a fantastically effective cycle of oxytocin and touch, so can our marriages. Once we have the urge to bond and we are physically comfortable, we can continue developing, moving on to emotional intimacy, just as an infant does.

When you stop to think about it, the only thing an infant has to offer is a deep, authentic, emotional connection with their caretakers. In other words, a child has to quickly learn how to get their own needs met while simultaneously making sure they are contributing to the well-being of their family members. Isn't that similar to what we need to do in a marriage?

In short, we are born with the natural instinct to connect, which is exactly what we need to survive. Yet somehow our culture encourages us to become "independent," thwarting our desire for intimacy and teaching us to control our emotions so thoroughly that they become unnoticeable, even to ourselves.

Think of young children who have no hesitation whatsoever about expressing their emotions. They cry when they're unhappy. They giggle when they're delighted. They express wonder when they're curious. Of course, to the horror of parents everywhere, they also throw screaming tantrums in the grocery store when they're furious at their parents for not buying them that candy bar in the checkout aisle.

Am I saying you should have a massive meltdown at the grocery store? No. But I do think there's something to be said for the pure, raw, unadulterated emotions of children. We don't have to mimic their behavior to learn from it.

My point is, as parents, we should encourage our children to feel their feelings but control their behavior. And as adults, we should excel at feeling our feelings while controlling our behavior.

Sadly, most of us try to control our emotions while claiming our behavior is out of our control. Argh. I don't think we are doing a good job of leading by example, nor are we making it easy to be happy ourselves.

It's time to stop denying our feelings, whether they are pleasant or not. As mature, healthy adults, we should be capable of acting in a reasonable manner regardless of how we feel. We should realize that our choices aren't limited to being ruled by our feelings or completely repressing them. It's sad that somewhere along the way, we accepted these as our only options. Whittling down our emotions to fit what's socially acceptable while swallowing the rest not only harms us, it's also incredibly destructive to our relationships.

You don't need to be an expert to see for yourself that people who grow up in emotionally healthy and expressive families have a much easier time forming healthy relationships as adults. That discussion is beyond the purview of this book, but if you're interested in learning more, I highly recommend reading *Attached: The New Science of Adult Attachment and How It Can Help You Find—and Keep—Love.*[27]

> Emotional intimacy is like anything else: the more we study and practice it, the better at it we'll be.

Emotional intimacy is like anything else: the more we study and practice it, the better at it we'll be.

What does that mean for you?

Even if you didn't grow up with healthy emotional intimacy, you can always start working on it now. Habits can be learned and unlearned.

When Emotional Intimacy Is Weaponized

We all have experience with emotional intimacy. What we don't all have in equal amounts is experience in noticing, articulating, and valuing our emotional experiences. If you are unconvinced, then remember that emotional intimacy, like every other kind of intimacy, can be wanted or unwanted, intentional or unintentional, joyous or embarrassing.

---

[27] Amir Levine MD and Rachel Heller, *Attached: The New Science of Adult Attachment and How It Can Help You Find–and Keep–Love*, PenguinRandomhouse. com (Penguin Adult HC/TR), https://www.penguinrandomhouse.com/ books/303069/attached-by-amir-levine-md-and-rachel-sf-heller-ma/.

If a man cried when he was a child and other boys made fun of him or, worse, if his father beat him for crying, that was emotional intimacy—even though it was most unwelcome.

It shouldn't be surprising that the most "unemotional" men often have had unpleasant experiences with emotional intimacy. It could reasonably be said that they learned the "lesson" so well that they even convinced themselves that they were imperturbable.

Of course, this goes for women too. It's not as if women don't have complicated feelings, histories, and baggage around expressing emotion. Plenty of women have been criticized or punished for honestly sharing their emotions.

It's hard to find a woman who hasn't heard things such as the following:

"You must be PMSing."
"Don't be such a bitch!"
"Why are you so angry?"
"You're too emotional."
"Do you really have to cry over spilled milk?"
"God, you're being hysterical!"

For a woman who is expressing her authentic emotions, comments like these can feel enormously invalidating. After hearing them repeatedly, they can make a person feel disconnected from their own emotions and inclined to bury them deep down just to keep the peace.

My editor has always been very emotionally forthcoming in her romantic relationships. After enduring a lot of heartbreak in college, she started seriously seeking a long-term relationship in her early twenties. She was looking for a partner with whom she could talk openly about her fears, about things as macro as world events (war, shootings, etc.) and as micro as the parts of the relationship that bothered her (the lack of shared friends, different bedtimes, etc.).

While she knew that talking openly was very important to her, what she didn't realize until we started working together on this book was that the conversations were really just the "packaging" for what she truly craved: emotional intimacy.

Every time she revealed something about what was important to her, it was in the hope that her loving partner would offer her a safe harbor from her fears by providing genuine comfort and support. In short, she wanted her partner to care about and respect her feelings while affording her the opportunity to do the same for him. She knew that the only way to have mutual health and happiness was if they were both able to share their feelings.

Unfortunately, she learned the hard way that some people find emotional intimacy to be troublesome rather than beneficial. At twenty-five, she was told by her boyfriend, "I'm looking for a partner, not a liability." His words shook her to the core. He had called her a liability simply because she'd dared to be honest about her needs and the parts of their relationship that required work.

Needless to say, they broke up!

I'm happy to report that in the years since that painful relationship, my editor has had several loving partners who appreciated the value she placed on emotional intimacy. It wasn't always because they were good at it; sometimes they wanted to learn from her how to be better! Now she's in her late thirties and head over heels in love with a guy with a natural flair for emotional intimacy. She has finally met her match.

Gotta Be Able to Let Go

I believe there's an emotional divorce and a legal divorce.

Some people go through an emotional divorce long before a legal one, while others remain emotionally connected long after legal documents are signed. In some cases, couples are able to maintain a positive emotional connection, which allows them to move forward as friends or cooperative co-parents. Sadly, there's more often a *negative* emotional connection that lingers, such as anger, resentment, or jealousy.

Being willing to open ourselves up to emotional intimacy is hugely important, but it's only half the battle. If we don't develop the ability to disconnect and move on, we can find ourselves being held prisoner by our emotional connections. This doesn't only occur via divorce; there are plenty of people who spend decades complaining about their highly dysfunctional marriage, yet they refuse to end things.

Why? The only answer has to be that somehow the negative connection is still better than no connection. Many people's only experiences with emotional intimacy have been negative, so they don't even realize there's a chance for anything different.

I can't emphasize this enough: we need to practice dealing with positive and negative emotional intimacy.

We need to learn that even though emotional intimacy can "backfire" on us, that we might not get the response we want, we're strong enough to cope with whatever happens. We have to remember that even happy couples fight and disappoint each other sometimes, even in big ways. The secret to surviving these disappointments is being able to nurture yourself in healthy ways until you're ready to address the problem with your partner. Think of boxers who take a few minutes to regroup alone in their corner but don't leave the ring just because they got hit. (Mind you, I am not a boxing fan because I can't stand fighting, but I do understand that rough times in marriage can be really ugly too. Remembering that there is a big payoff for each of you if you stay in the "ring" together might be the visualization you need to see things through.)

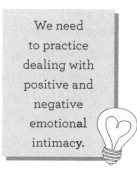

We need to practice dealing with positive and negative emotional intimacy.

If you're someone who has learned to flee rather than risk being emotionally vulnerable, ask your head (not your scared heart) whether your partner is reasonably trustworthy. If they are, perhaps you can make an agreement with your partner that your relationship will be a training ground of sorts. Give each other permission to make mistakes but promise to follow them with amends.

I seek this kind of agreement from my clients all the time. Bringing emotions to the forefront can quickly make things messy, complicated, heated, and hard. I keep my clients "in the ring" by asking them to agree to a "divorce moratorium" for 90 to 180 days (barring any unforeseen circumstances, of course). It's not reasonable to expect that anyone is going to willingly be emotionally vulnerable if they think their partner might file for divorce the next day.

Don't be afraid to ask for whatever safety parameters you might need. It's a great first step in learning to trust not only your partner but also yourself.

The truth is, no matter who we are or how we were raised, we live in a culture that generally doesn't value the kind of emotional intimacy that is healthy, consensual, and desired. We're all encouraged to stay busy, stuff our schedules full, and pretend that spending a few minutes commenting on our friends' social media posts is enough to keep us connected to our friends. It has become an unusual practice to engage in a long heart-to-heart conversation over an in-person cup of coffee, which is a huge loss for all of us.

> Don't be afraid to ask for whatever safety parameters you might need. It's a great first step in learning to trust not only your partner but also yourself.

The kind of emotional intimacy that we need—the kind that keeps us living longer and feeling happier—requires time to grow, develop, and flourish. It takes more than sharing the high points of our life. But making the effort really *is* worth it. It helps us to not only be better partners but also better people. We are more attuned to the people around us. We have more empathy. We become better able to drop into our own emotions, to be honest with ourselves about what we want and what we need—even when it comes to sexy stuff.

This is where it's so easy for marriages to get off track. If we start "phoning it in," as we do with our friendships, giving our relationships only the bare minimum of emotional intimacy, it's highly likely that our sexual intimacy will suffer too. I mean, it's kinda hard to be a good and generous lover when you're focused on keeping all your other feelings under wraps. (Yes, I know sex can be a good stress reliever, but speaking from experience, being someone's stress relief isn't the same thing as having sexy fun with them!)

To clarify, I don't believe that emotional intimacy is required before a couple can have great sexual intimacy. But I know beyond a shadow of a doubt that having great emotional intimacy can improve even the hottest sexy fun. After all, anatomy can be responsible for sexual intimacy, but emotional intimacy provides the insights necessary to give pleasure beyond mere orgasm.

Again, this is just another example of how the different kinds of intimacy are interrelated. A couple may come to my office thinking that sex is the problem in their relationship—that if they could just have more sex, or better sex, or more orgasms, they'd have the union of their dreams. But it quickly becomes apparent to all of us that there's more to it.

So let's turn our attention to the third kind of intimacy.

It's time for a sexy awakening!

Tantalizing Takeaways

- Emotional intimacy is like anything else: the more we study and practice it, the better at it we'll be.

- An easy way to recognize your emotional intimacy with a partner is to ask yourself if sharing something (whether good or bad) with your partner helps you to feel better. If your answer is "yes"—awesome, you're on your way to an even deeper level of emotional intimacy. If it's "no" or "maybe," you might want to revisit this chapter as well as Intimacy Practice #5 (page 203).

- Even though emotional intimacy can backfire, the secret to surviving these disappointments is being able to nurture yourself in healthy ways until you're ready to address the problem with your partner.

XOXO

Sometimes It Is Sexual

Sexual intimacy occurs when our sexual body parts—or anything relating to our erotic selves, truths, secrets, fears, frustrations, or challenges—are involved or exposed. The level of such intimacy varies depending on the amount of vulnerability involved.

Believe it or not, sexual intimacy isn't just about sex. Yes, there is sexual intimacy when people engage in sexual acts with others. But we also have sexual intimacy with our gynecologist or proctologist. Sexual intimacy doesn't always require physical intimacy; phone sex and cybersex are sexually intimate too, as are conversations about sex and hearing other people have sex. In this chapter, we'll reveal some surprising truths about sexual intimacy—including its ugly side.

> Sexual intimacy occurs when our sexual body parts— or anything relating to our erotic selves, truths, secrets, fears, frustrations, or challenges— are involved or exposed.

***

One of my favorite examples of nonphysical sexual intimacy comes from a most surprising couple.

Ted and Tracy were virgins when they married shortly after high school. Over forty years later, the couple would tell anyone who would listen that love and their faith had gotten them through it all. They were both very traditional, religious people, active in their church and devoted to their children. While they were fun-loving people, they never swore.

Sadly, their marriage was interrupted by cancer. As Tracy's time on Earth grew shorter, she slept in a hospital bed in the living room with Ted next to her in his recliner.

One morning, as Ted attempted to slip out of the room without waking Tracy, she called him over to her bed. She had so little breath left that she had to ask him to lean closer because she had something to tell him. With trepidation, Ted leaned down, fearing he was about to hear her last words.

He steeled himself with a deep breath before saying, "I'm here, honey."

Her voice barely above a whisper, eyes sparkling with an energy Ted hadn't seen in months, Tracy said, "You wanna f**k?"

Ted was so shocked he almost fell over! He didn't know whether to laugh or cry, so he did both. Despite her frailty, Tracy was almost radiant, so pleased was she by having playfully shocked and surprised this man who thought he knew her so well.

Within two weeks, Tracy was gone. Ted was alone but for his memories. Of all their good times, all the wonderful years they shared together, that unexpected moment of spicy humor became one of Ted's most cherished memories. Tracy's simple yet outlandish comment celebrated the special intimacy that was theirs and theirs alone.

Yes, sexual intimacy certainly includes having sex. But that's not the whole story. Even though Tracy was too weak to actually engage in physical sexy fun with her husband, her "You wanna f**k?" comment was such a beautiful, completely irreverent example of how embracing sexual intimacy as love can serve to bring a couple closer, even in the midst of great pain. When we honor sexual intimacy as meaningful rather than banal, it creates an extremely powerful, rewarding connection.

When Waiting Is Harmful

Sharing our erotic truths, secrets, fears, frustrations, challenges, and yes, even dirty jokes with another person is sexual intimacy, but when sexual intimacy involves touch or pleasure intended to create erotic arousal or orgasmic pleasure, I describe that as *high-level* sexual intimacy.

This can be an important distinction, especially for couples who choose to wait to consummate their marriage until after they've exchanged vows. I've met far too many couples who studiously avoided all sexual intimacy, including conversations about their desires, until their honeymoon, only to then discover that they have vastly different expectations. One might imagine quiet, lights-off lovemaking once or twice a week, while the other has so much pent-up desire that they want sexy fun morning, noon, and night!

It's no different than agreeing to go out for a fancy dinner after the theater, only to discover that one of you thought that meant a four-course French meal and the other was excited for counter seats at the hot new sushi bar. Relationships stand a greater chance of success when we learn to address each person's expectations in advance rather than presuming that your imaginations are in sync. This is no different when it comes to sexual intimacy. One's intention to be a virgin at the wedding should *never* preclude having extremely forthright conversations in advance about each person's vision of the role sexual intimacy will play in the marriage.

> When sexual intimacy involves touch or pleasure intended to create erotic arousal or orgasmic pleasure, I describe that as high-level sexual intimacy.

Let's look at it from a completely different perspective.

But Nothing Happened

Meet Bob and Carla had been married for twenty-eight years when I met them. They loved each other and were committed to making their marriage work.

However, they had gotten mired in an unending argument about one of Bob's coworkers. Carla was incredibly unhappy; she felt that Bob's friendship with his female coworker—let's call her Eleanor—was inappropriate, even threatening. Carla believed Bob when he said he hadn't had sex with Eleanor, but she was still jealous. Even without sex, Carla felt Bob's close relationship with this woman was "cheating."

For the nine months leading up to their first session with me, Bob and Carla had been stuck in an endless cycle, arguing about this relationship. Bob swore that this was not an affair, that Eleanor was simply a friend. He was adamant that he had not broken any of his vows. By the time I met him, he was angry and defensive. In his mind, Carla was unjustified in accusing him of doing anything wrong. He strongly believed he should be allowed to continue his relationship with Eleanor even with Carla being bothered.

Bob admitted that he spoke with Eleanor about his marriage, his relationship with Carla—even the struggles they'd been having in their sex life. But he felt this was perfectly reasonable since Eleanor also spoke to him about her husband and their issues. He said it was nice to get a female perspective, probably even good for his marriage, because he felt it would help him understand Carla better.

Carla was of two minds. On the one hand, she believed Bob that he had not gotten physical with Eleanor. But on the other, there was still something about the relationship that felt dangerous and disrespectful to her, though she couldn't figure out why. She was miserable and heartbroken. She wondered if she was being "crazy."

Do you see what I see in that story? Do you see how Bob and his coworker shared emotional intimacy as friends—but also sexual intimacy because they talked about their sex lives? Do you understand that sexual intimacy doesn't require engaging in sexual activity together?

> Sexual intimacy occurs when our sexual body parts—or anything relating to our erotic selves, truths, secrets, fears, frustrations, or challenges—are involved or exposed.

When you stop to think about it, it becomes clear that the conversations Bob was having with Eleanor contained all the ingredients of sexual intimacy: Sexual intimacy occurs when our sexual body parts—or anything relating to our erotic selves, truths, secrets, fears, frustrations, or challenges—are involved or exposed.

Yep, you read that right: you can experience sexual intimacy without ever touching another person.

Sexual Intimacy Surrounds Us

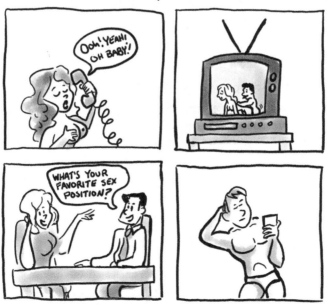

Sexual intimacy is also the following:

- Participating in phone sex
- Partaking in any type of sexual activity
- Sending an erotic photo, poem, story, or video
- Watching porn together
- Watching someone have sex
- Engaging in self-pleasure
- Watching webcam performers
- Undergoing a pelvic or prostate exam
- Reading sexy letters or notes[28]
- Talking about sexual issues with friends, family, doctors, other professionals, or even a platonic friend (read: Eleanor)
- Being pregnant—because obviously there's been sexual intimacy! (That's actually why a lot of teenagers feel uncomfortable when their moms are pregnant. That baby bump is a reminder of their parents' sexuality, and most kids don't like to be that sexually intimate with their parents!)
- Engaging in oral sex[29]
- Engaging in anal sex
- Listening to someone having sex
- Experiencing rape or sexual assault*

*When Intimacy Is Ugly

Trigger Warning: I want to say something about the last item in the list above because it's important. Our first thought when we hear the word *intimacy* may be that it is something sweet and good. But intimacy

---

[28] Funny story: my mom found out my boyfriend and I were having sex in high school because his mom read a card I had given him—and then she told my mom!

[29] Can you see how asking Bill Clinton if he experienced sexual intimacy with Monica Lewinsky might have been a much more effective question?

can also be ugly. Also, as we've seen, intimacy does not require or imply consent.

In the years that I've been teaching the 5 Kinds of Intimacy, I've gotten plenty of pushback about associating intimacy with rape. I have listened carefully, discussed it with other experts in the field, and spent a lot of time challenging myself on this point.

Please don't think I take this lightly. This is serious to me personally, as well as professionally. I was a trained volunteer rape crisis advocate even before I started law school. I've witnessed firsthand the horror that remains after a sexual assault, and I've cried with more survivors than I can count. I don't pretend to know everything, but I know that being sexually assaulted is very different than being violently mugged.

Years ago, the widely accepted belief was that calling rape a *sexual act* somehow implied fault or consent by the victim. So rape was categorized instead as an *act of violence*. The thinking was that this would ensure rape victims did not feel "less than" victims of other crimes.

But failing to acknowledge the sexual aspects of rape had unintended consequences. Rape victims were now grouped in with the victims of other acts of physical violence, defined as "(A) an assault or other infliction or threat of infliction of death or bodily harm on an individual; or (B) damage to, or destruction of, real or personal property."[30]

As any survivor of sexual assault knows, it's just not the same. Of course, different crimes violate us by forcing different kinds of unwanted intimacy upon us, but rape is unique in that the victim also experiences forced *sexual* intimacy. The law's lumping together of rape and physical violence caused even more trauma for rape victims because it failed to recognize one particular harm inflicted. In truth, survivors of sexual assault need specific support and understanding in order to heal and recover.

---

[30] "Definition: Act of Physical Violence from 40 USC § 5104(a)(1)," Legal Information Institute, https://www.law.cornell.edu/definitions/uscode.php?width=840&height=800&iframe=true&def_id=40-USC-1390921591-2033562886.

Fortunately, the scientific and legal community started listening. The studies have finally caught up to what rape survivors have been telling us all along: Rape is different.[31] Sexual trauma is not the same thing as a physical blow. While rape may well be about power, aggression, or violence rather than the rapist's sexual desire, the reality is that the "weapon" used is sexual intimacy. Failing to address the specific impact of this crime is to deny the survivors the respect and help they deserve.

I find it *empowering*, rather than disempowering, to address sexual traumas differently than other violent crimes. By doing so, we can provide a better framework for addressing the unique harm suffered by survivors of rape and sexual assault. We can address the shame they often feel that is distinctly different from that of other crime victims. This supports my own definition of sexual intimacy. To deny that rape is a form, albeit an ugly form, of sexual intimacy is to ignore the very aspect that distinguishes it from other assaults. Regardless of intention, it *feels* sexual to the victim. Not in a pleasurable way, of course—but sexually intimate in a horrible, painful, traumatizing way.

I want to acknowledge that it can sometimes be especially hard for people who have experienced rape, assault, or other forms of trauma to enjoy sexual intimacy, even with their beloved partners. The topic deserves its own book; I can't possibly give it the attention it deserves here. But I hope to offer some simple, small steps to guide you toward a new version of sexy fun that feels safe to *you*. I'll share ideas for exercises in which you are the one in charge; you get to determine when and how it's okay for your partner to touch you—or specify that *only you* do the touching. (Please don't miss the Just Say NO! Intimacy Practice later on in this book.)

---

[31] Hane Htut Maung, "A Dilemma in Rape Crisis and a Contribution from Philosophy," Nature News (Nature Publishing Group, April 8, 2021), https://www.nature.com/articles/s41599-021-00769-y.

I promise that joyful, fulfilling sexual intimacy is available to you too. No matter what you have survived, your past trauma does not have to rob you of that. You *deserve* to have—and I want to help you get to—a place where sexual intimacy feels not just enjoyable but also empowering.

***

I'm very used to people assuming that they know what sexual intimacy is because they believe it's so patently obvious. That's why I shared Bob and Carla's story. Their situation shows that sexual intimacy is more nuanced—more complex—than one might assume.

Some people firmly believe that talking about sex outside of one's romantic relationship is the equivalent of having an affair. Others are equally convinced that talking about sex is completely different than *having* sex and that even married people should be able to talk about it with whomever they choose.

While you ponder your thoughts on the matter, let's consider the role sexual intimacy plays in relationships that *aren't* romantic.

I'd like to introduce you to Paul.

Sexual Intimacy: It's Not Always What You Think

Paul grew up in a very loving, tight-knit family. His parents were good people who loved their children and tried to do everything they could to make sure their kids would grow up to be productive professionals with their own happy families.

Paul adored everything about his parents and other family members . . . except for one thing. They were very religious, which, for them, meant they were adamantly opposed to homosexuality. In fact, Paul's parents believed homosexuality is a sin that guarantees someone an eternity in hell.

This was problematic for Paul because even though he had been trying to resist being gay since he was twelve years old, by the time I met him at thirty-five, he had realized that being gay is not optional; it's simply who he is.

A couple of years ago, Paul, being the devoted son that he is, decided that the fact that he is gay didn't mean he had to indulge his desires. Though he was sexually active for most of his twenties, he felt so much guilt that he didn't enjoy sex anyway. He thought that would make it easy for him to be celibate. With that mindset, he would spend the next two years avoiding sex. He tried to convince himself that he could enjoy living alone forever. He worked hard to give up his dream of having a spouse, kids, and a "family life."

He didn't tell his parents or siblings any of this. Every time he talked with them or met them for family dinners, his siblings asked if he was dating anyone or when he was going to get married. They teased him about his age, but no one ever even *hinted* he might be gay. Paul's secret was truly a secret.

You probably aren't surprised to learn that Paul's attempted celibacy did not prove to be a realistic option. In fact, what brought Paul to me was the fact that he had met the man he thought could be his forever love, yet he was miserable. He hated hiding such an important part of his life from his family.

Long story long: My work with Paul involved his recognizing that the 5 Kinds of Intimacy apply even to his relationship with his parents. He came to realize that—*wow*—while he'd never expected he would need to have sexual intimacy with his *parents,* of all people, he actually did.

That's not to say that he needed to have sex with his parents! Rather, he needed them to see him as a man, as a sexual, romantic being with human needs and desires. In old-fashioned parlance, Paul wanted to come out of the closet. To do so, he would have to be sexually intimate with his parents, whether they liked it or not.

SOMETIMES IT IS SEXUAL

Now do you understand why sexual intimacy is not just about having sex? It can be so complicated, yet it's an integral part of a safe, healthy, happy relationship.

With that in mind, let's return to Carla and Bob's dilemma. Who do you think is right?

Do you think it's okay for Bob to have a female friend with whom he shares details about his marriage? Or do you think that relationship should be terminated?

Take a minute to think about why you feel the way you do. Can you come up with "guidelines for future use" for you and your partner—a way to decide what's okay and what's not okay for your relationship? (I'd be very interested in hearing your thoughts, so if you'd like to share them with me, please email me at beth@darlingway.com!)

Would you like to hear *my* thoughts?

I believe that when it comes to determining if an activity qualifies as "cheating," the deciding factor is whether or not secrecy is involved. If Bob is having lunch on a regular basis with Eleanor but is subtly or overtly keeping that from Carla, that raises some alarms for me.

> I believe that when it comes to determining if an activity qualifies as "cheating," the deciding factor is whether or not secrecy is involved.

On the other hand, if he has lunch with her regularly but answers Carla's calls in the middle of lunch with "Hey! Eleanor says hi!" I don't believe he is doing anything improper. In other words, if there is no pretense, no sneaking around, and Bob is happy to introduce the two women and share stories with Carla about his coworker without any sense of shame or concern, I think that kind of openness indicates that this work relationship doesn't pose a threat to the marriage.

Another thing I look for is if someone is feeling guilty. Then I want to know why. Some of us feel guilty simply for existing, but if it's about the relationship, there might be underlying romantic feelings that could be problematic.

My personal belief is that we are all better for having friends from different backgrounds, of different genders, with different beliefs and experiences. That's how we learn, how we grow.

I have sympathy for men because it is uncommon for them to discuss their sexual problems with other men. Assuming that Bob is truly faithful to Carla, it would be perfectly reasonable for him to be seeking advice from his friends about how to improve his marriage. It's also reasonable for him to think that he might receive more pertinent advice on the matter from another married woman, who can better empathize with Carla than his buddies can.

> My personal belief is that we are all better for having friends from different backgrounds, of different genders, with different beliefs and experiences. That's how we learn, how we grow.

I think that sexualizing all relationships between men and women is a harmful practice. While *When Harry Met Sally* is a great movie, I don't agree with the basic premise. I firmly believe men and women *can* just be friends and that their friendships can add serious value to their relationships. Harry needed to know that women are really good at faking orgasms, but his male friends probably didn't know any better than he did! (Of course, I hope the only fake orgasms in your life are those enacted for fun in very nonsexual situations! Only real orgasms in your sex life, please!)

Curious about how Bob and Carla are now? I'm happy to report that Bob really wasn't hiding anything from Carla. He really was just looking for help because their relationship had been miserably strained. In their work with me, we spent a lot of time helping them reestablish the emotional intimacy they had lost. Once we'd accomplished that, Carla felt confident that Bob's other friendships, even with Eleanor, were a blessing, not a threat. Fortunately, Eleanor had no designs on Bob either, which was great because the work Bob did with me not only improved his marriage but also hers! Yep. They continue to be friends, but now they have Carla's blessing. The cherry on top is that when Carla's upset with Bob these days, she'll often call Eleanor and ask her to help set him straight!

As for Paul, I wish I could tell you his family opened their hearts to him after his disclosure. But they didn't. Sadly, he has very little contact with them now, which has caused him tremendous pain. However, he finds comfort in the knowledge that he did his best to maintain a healthy relationship with them. He realizes that no relationship is worth sacrificing himself. Despite this loss, Paul is able to take pride in the fact that he has established a healthy level of *self*-intimacy in each of the five areas, which has given him the confidence to create a very healthy marriage with the love of his life.

The End of Sex—and the Beginning of Sexy Fun

So, we've talked a lot about other people in this chapter. Let's get back to you, shall we?

Because I bet you're wondering: *So shouldn't we just have more sex?*

Great question.

Let's talk about sex.

I've spoken with thousands of women about their sex lives. Here's how the conversation usually goes when the woman is married (even if she loves her husband!):

Me: "When was the last time you had sex?"

Her: "Last week. Or the week before, maybe."

Me: "Did you orgasm?"

Her: "Ummm . . . no."

Me: "Was it fun?"

Her: (long pause) "Not really."

It makes me want to bang my head against the wall! I cringe every time I think about how hurt their husbands would be to hear this. Yet because they *aren't* hearing it, they aren't doing anything differently, which is why their wives aren't excited about having more sex, *duh!*

These couples are having what I call *BMS* (boring married sex—which doesn't actually require marriage, *BTW* [by the way]).

Here's how you know if you're having boring married sex: Your sex life is a rotation through a few positions, moves, or techniques that have proved efficient over time. Each of you pretty much knows what to do and what to expect. It's familiar, predictable, and comfortable. It's not exciting, surprising, thrilling, or memorable.

But hey, while BMS isn't the passionate, exciting sexy fun I wish for you, at least it's a big improvement over a sexless marriage—which around 25 percent of couples are experiencing.

Plus, the fact that you're reading this book means you're open to new ideas. So I think you're poised to amp up your sexual intimacy in a powerfully pleasurable way!

> If your sex life is a rotation through the same few positions, moves, or techniques, you're having *BMS*. Each of you pretty much knows what to do and what to expect. It's familiar, predictable, and comfortable. It's not exciting, surprising, thrilling, or memorable.

So many couples are stuck in a rut because they don't know what else to do. But I'm going to help you use curiosity, kindness, and generosity to create endlessly fun ways to play together in the bedroom (and other rooms too!).

Let's start with what is generally meant by the word *sex* these days:

sex = erection & orgasm (his)

This is why I refuse to settle for *sex* anymore.

I want *sexy fun*. In other words, I want exciting, enticing, exhilarating, erotically charged pleasure.

On the other hand, sometimes I want *sexy love*, a term I use to refer to more solemn lovemaking sessions, ones in which the mood is more serious than lighthearted.

Words matter. They create expectations in our minds as well as our partner's. The more specifically intentional we are with our word choices, the more likely we are to get what we want.

Which brings me to this question: What do you want?

Please note the following facts about sexy fun and sexy love:

- Sexy fun, by definition, means that both people have to enjoy it. (Yay for consent!)
- Neither sexy fun nor sexy love require erections or orgasm, though they can certainly take place.
- Sexy fun isn't goal-oriented other than its being fun for all.
- The only objective of sexy love is for a couple to envelop each other in the pleasure of being loved.
- Sexy fun and sexy love don't necessarily end just because someone orgasmed.
- Whether it's sexy fun or sexy love, the only true "foreplay" is shaving your legs or whatever you do to *get ready* for the occasion because everything you do to arouse, tease, pleasure, and play is pure sexy fun or sexy love!

Both sexy fun and sexy love can be as lighthearted or solemn as you both desire at any given moment. Personally and professionally, including in this book, I use the terms interchangeably.

Now, if you're thinking that having sexy fun is code for "girls gone wild" or the male equivalent, let me be clear: Sexy fun is whatever *you* find erotically enjoyable and entertaining.

Sexy fun is whatever you find erotically enjoyable and entertaining.

Some people think making love with the lights on is great sexy fun. Others want to run naked through the woods together. Quite simply, there are at least as many ways to have sexy fun as there are humans on this planet. Don't worry about what *others* are doing unless you're looking for new ideas to consider for yourself.

To give you a sense of how easy it is to get out of the BMS rut, here are several easy-peasy methods that have worked wonders for my clients:

- Make eye contact during sexy fun (not necessarily all the time, but periodically). You can even pause for a few seconds of eye gazing. You won't believe how powerful it is until you try it! If your partner likes to keep their eyes closed during sexy stuff, don't be afraid to ask them to open them and look at you.

- Start sexy fun by teasing, touching, or talking about your desires way before bedtime—certainly before you enter your bedroom. This creates anticipation and gives your partner a chance to adjust their expectations for the evening.

- Find new places to have sexy fun in your house. Or yard. Or garage. Or office. You don't have to go to a hotel to enjoy hotel-sex-level excitement!

- Use your words. Tell your partner how you feel. What you want. How much you like their body, or what they're doing, or what you're doing to them. Make slow, deliciously sensual love sometimes. Other times, enjoy a quickie in the garage before you go out to dinner. Take chances, wear outrageous costumes or racy lingerie, read erotica—whatever it takes to keep both of you engaged.

If you're having sex without having fun, you're basically eating flavorless ice cream. Sure, it feels nice to swallow something cold and creamy on a hot day (did I actually say that?!), but why would you deprive yourself of the added pleasure of flavor?[32] Doesn't a delectable, sweet cream with strawberries or a decadent rocky road sound perfect right now? *Mmmm!*

By the way, when I say *BMS*, you might think I'm talking about missionary sex, but I'm not at all. (Missionary position is generally defined as a man lying on a woman, face to face). I'm well aware that missionary sex is often the butt of the joke. "You only do it missionary?" someone might say, teasing their friend. "Boring!" Even the name doesn't exactly ooze sex appeal. When we imagine missionaries out in the jungle, handing out gospel tracts, we don't exactly envision them banging one another senseless under the mango trees!

Yet, frankly, I love missionary sex. You can make eye contact a lot more easily than you can in, say, doggy-style sex. (But that's not to say doggy style isn't great fun too!)

But back to the missionary position. Looking into your partner's eyes while making love can be an easy way to continue enjoying your sexy pleasure while also adding a component of emotional intimacy. After all, there's really no place to hide when you're clenched together, face to face. This creates a fantastic vulnerability, which can amp up the erotic charge between you exponentially. Trust me: vulnerability can be *hot*.

All You Have to Do Is Dream . . .[33]

I've gotta talk to you about fantasies for a minute.

---

[32] It's amazing how many times I attempted to include an emoji in this book but my editor wouldn't let me! Sigh. Just pretend there's a blushing smiley face here, followed by an eggplant . . . ;)

[33] If you want to listen to this wonderful oldies song, check out the Everly Brothers singing "All I Have to Do Is Dream" on YouTube! https://www.youtube.com/watch?v=tbU3zdAgiX8.

A lot of therapists say, "It's okay to think about other sexual fantasies while you're having sex with your partner." Hmmm. Let's think about this for a minute.

I'm all in favor of people having hot, sexy fantasies. But who wants to have sex with someone who's mentally having sex with somebody else? *Not me,* that's for damn sure!

That's not to say that I don't encourage my clients to enjoy fantasies in their sex life; it's just that I want them to do it in a way that brings them closer to their partner, not further away from them.

Think about it. If you're fantasizing about someone else during sexy fun, you're mentally escaping the sexy fun your body is actually having. That seems kind of hurtful, doesn't it? Your partner is right there, offering themself to you for mutual pleasure. There's such a great opportunity for a steamy connection since their desire for you is evident. But you're thinking about someone else? I can't imagine how that could possibly be good for a relationship.

Wanna know what *is* good for a relationship? Sharing your fantasies. Letting your fantasies elevate the sexy fun for both of you.

Here's an example of what I mean. Just for the sake of science, let's say I have a huge celebrity crush on Ryan Gosling. He makes me melt from the inside out. I've seen all his movies, some more than once, and I think he's so damn sexy. I mean, how could I watch *The Notebook* and *not* fall head over heels in love with that guy?

But how can my fantasy of being with Ryan Gosling possibly help my relationship with my partner? How do I share it with my partner without intimidating them or pissing them off?

Well, given that most of us have at least one or two celebrity crushes, the first thing we should agree on is that it doesn't mean our relationship is "less than" or that we are going to cheat. Or even that we *want* to cheat! In fact, I think you can learn a lot about your partner and even improve your relationship by talking with them about both of your celebrity crushes.

I say this because when we are crushing on a celebrity, it's not usually all that personal. Sounds crazy, but it's true. I don't know Ryan Gosling in real life. I know how I *think* he might behave in certain situations—okay, how he behaved in certain *roles*—but I don't know the guy from Adam. What I do know is that his on-screen persona turns me on. Seriously. Just the thought of him makes me want to turn on the TV!

My favorite Ryan Gosling movie is *Crazy, Stupid Love.* Ryan is terrific in his role as Jacob, a smooth-talking, impeccably dressed player who appears wildly confident—but who is, deep down, as insecure as everyone else. Emma Stone does a wonderful job playing Hannah, the "normal," down-to-earth woman Jacob falls in love with when he finally tires of all his one-night stands.

Jacob's persistence in chasing her, his sexual confidence, and his sincere desire for her draw Hannah in despite her fears that he's "out of her league." Sure, it's just another version of "when the wild boy meets the right girl, he'll be good forevermore." We've all heard *that* before! But I can't help wanting to be the "right" one . . . especially for Ryan Gosling.

So what if I told my partner that I had a crush on Ryan? And, what if, instead of feeling hurt or insecure, he took it as an opportunity to have some Ryan Gosling-inspired sexy fun with me?

"This is what Ryan would do," my partner might say. Or "Remember the part in *Crazy, Stupid Love* when he takes his shirt off?" Then he might do a little striptease inspired by the scene in which Jacob seduces Hannah. (Give me a second while I fan myself, please.)

This is one example of how we can incorporate our fantasies into our sex lives without hurting each other, without taking ourselves out of the moment. My guy can rest easy knowing that it's not that I actually want Ryan Gosling in my bed (though I'm not saying I'd complain about it!); it's that I want to be wanted by the hot guy. I want to feel special, like the way Jacob makes Hannah feel. I want to experience the energy of an unexpected new romance. These are all things my partner can bring into the bedroom for some mutual sexy fun.

Sexual Intimacy Is for Everyone

You wouldn't believe how many people think happy, healthy sexual intimacy isn't for them. They believe it's a pipe dream, a fantasy, something they just can't have.

Alternately, some people think sexual intimacy is *all* they can achieve. They may even have a committed partner, but to them, if it's not sexual, it's not intimacy.

When people experience sexual intimacy in a vacuum, it's like fast food: It might scratch an itch, but it doesn't sustain good feelings for long. Who doesn't love a nice greasy box of french fries every once in a while? But it doesn't take long for us to crave something a bit more fulfilling.

So how do you know if you're in a vacuum? When there's nothing to say to each other after you've had sex. When there's no desire to touch each other post-orgasm. When there's no interest in spending time together other than to participate in sexy stuff.

When couples tell me they never make eye contact during sex, that's another indication that they may not be enjoying the kind of sexy fun I want for them. Awareness is huge. Being present is huge. When you make eye contact, you have to be present *in that moment with that person.* It's a recognition of your physical, sexual, and emotional intimacy.

One common issue for many people is that even while they are engaging in sexual activity, they may be subconsciously avoiding going "all in." I see this often in clients who have been sexually traumatized, many of whom have very valid reasons to approach sex with wariness. But this reticence isn't always informed by sexual trauma. I also see it in people who have hang-ups about sex for other reasons. Maybe they were raised in a religion where sex was shamed or stigmatized. Perhaps (like Paul) they come from a family that held damaging beliefs around sex or sexual preferences. Maybe they absorbed other messaging, such as that from a former partner who told them they weren't very good at sex or didn't look good naked, or some other whisper that continually haunts them.

Regardless of their reasons, when these people get into romantic relationships, they'll often tell me things such as the following:

- I can't orgasm with a partner.
- Sure, they're great, but I'm just not feeling it (just like it was with my last five partners).
- I'm not really interested in sex.
- They're so demanding that it's a total turnoff.
- I feel kind of floaty during sex.
- I just can't stand how messy it is.

Then they unknowingly add insult to injury. Rather than recognizing and dealing with why things don't feel right, they just live with their discomfort. Over time, they gradually become even more disengaged from their sexual experiences, their partners, and themselves. Some disassociate so completely that their partners complain that they just "lie there like a dead fish." Ouch! That's pretty awful for all concerned.

So what do I suggest for couples who find themselves in this, *ahem*, position?

Easy. I suggest they work on emotional and spiritual self-intimacy.

I want them to discover if they've got any "blockages" for which we can find work-arounds or start building a tunnel through.

Again, until we know ourselves, we're not going to make ourselves available for others to know. When each party in a relationship has a reasonable understanding of their own emotional and spiritual response to sexual intimacy, then we can work on improving their relationship.

I know this may sound tough, but really, it's great news!

It means it's not a hopeless situation. It means it may not be a sexual problem—even if a person has gone more than forty years without enjoying sex despite trying every vibrator on the market. It means that they can stop trying to fake it. They can relax. Sure, they've got issues, but we all do. They're entitled to take some time to diagnose their maladies and heal themselves, just as if they had the flu.

Isn't it exciting to know that none of us has to settle for less-than-sexy fun anymore?

Oh, you know what goes really well with sexy fun? Actually, what goes really well with almost everything in life? How about a little romantic intimacy? *Oh là là*!

If I just made you want to puff out your chest and sing "Macho Man," hold on a minute! Romantic intimacy probably doesn't mean what you think it does. Romance is an ingredient that some people think is optional, but it's really like salt: It adds flavor while teasing our senses, creating a desire for more. And it doesn't improve just bland things; even something as delightfully sweet as chocolate is more delectable with a touch of sea salt!

Tantalizing Takeaways

- You can experience sexual intimacy without actually touching another person!
- Being sexually intimate doesn't require or guarantee emotional intimacy.
- Sexual intimacy without any romantic intimacy is a leading cause of BMS.

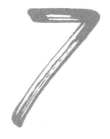

Go Ahead, Be a Raging Romantic

Romantic intimacy is when energy, ambiance, excitement, and/or surprise elevates an experience from ordinary to extraordinary. It's a picnic under the Eiffel Tower versus a picnic in your backyard. It may or may not occur in conjunction with sexual intimacy. In this chapter, we'll discover the ways in which our cultural idea of "romance"—spending money on luxury items such as flowers, jewelry, etc.—is different from romantic intimacy. Romantic intimacy encompasses so much more.

> Romantic intimacy is when energy, ambiance, excitement, and/or surprise elevates an experience from ordinary to extraordinary.

***

Romance is another one of those words that, like *intimacy*, gets tossed around willy-nilly. Most of us never stop to analyze it. It's not like we're going to be tested on it, so we just take it for granted, like the air we breathe.

The problem is we've internalized the culturally accepted idea of romance from books, movies, and oh-so-many ads (TV, magazines, billboards, mailers). We accept the prevailing pretense that romance is inherent in objects and events—sunsets, symphonies, candlelit dinners, and boxes of fancy chocolates.

Before we can use the word *romance*, we have to clarify its meaning. I believe that to do so, it's helpful to seek a historical perspective to decipher the nuances and subtext. Hallmark shouldn't get to rewrite the dictionary!

Ready for a little time travel with me? Let's go back to the Romantic period. This was an eighteenth-century literary, artistic, and philosophical movement defined by five core characteristics:

1. Interest in people's shared experiences
2. Strong senses, emotions, and feelings
3. Awe of nature
4. Celebration of the individual
5. Importance of imagination

Isn't that interesting? The way we currently use the word *romantic* is not in keeping with its original meaning! We have this idea that romance is confined to sexual relationships when really the word encompasses so much.

Romance is a sense of awe and wonder, a refusal to take the world for granted. Romantics celebrate even the smallest delights, grateful for their vast range of emotions.

That's what romantic intimacy is all about. It's about opening ourselves up to the world, not just buying chocolates in heart-shaped boxes.

Wait, let me say it more clearly: Romance is not just sappy stuff. And it's *not* just for women.

> Romance is a sense of awe and wonder, a refusal to take the world for granted. Romantics celebrate even the smallest delights, grateful for their vast range of emotions.

It's time to reclaim romance from the schmaltzy, saccharine narrative we've been given so that we can return to its roots—roots that can be sexy, surprising, unexpected, exciting, even extraordinary.

Since most men aren't used to thinking about what's "romantic" to them, I often ask them about it in a different way: "What do you think is hot?" Suddenly, they'll have lots of romantic ideas! This is perfect because the two words *actually mean the same thing*. What's "hot" isn't a different version of what's "romantic." It *is* romance—because romance is so much bigger, sexier, and more thrilling than the bill of goods we've been sold.

In fact, I learned this lesson the "hard" way (wink, wink).

Different Strokes (ahem) for Different Folks

A few years ago, I was talking to a guy I had just met. We'd been speaking on the phone for a couple of hours, enjoying getting to know each other. Obviously, my work is a bit unusual, so he was quite intrigued. I didn't mind his questions, even when they were personal.

So we were talking about a lot of sexy stuff that night. We were flirting, teasing each other. None of this was out of the ordinary for me. It was easy, lighthearted banter. I certainly wasn't feeling a high level of emotional intimacy. I wasn't being any more vulnerable with him than I am with the students in my *How to Blow His Mind While Loving His Body* workshop.

But this guy was eating it up (pun totally intended). He was a fifty-something man who didn't talk about sexual stuff with anybody, let alone a woman he'd just met. It felt highly emotionally intimate to him—something that, at the time, I failed to recognize.

After a few hours, we hung up with promises to get dinner together soon. Moments later, I got a text from him. I smiled as I opened it, expecting a sweet message about how glad he was to have met me. What I received instead still makes me shake my head in disbelief!

The very proper, conservative, suit-wearing man had sent me a pic of . . . *ahem* . . . his *pride and joy*, if you know what I mean.!

It takes a lot to shock me, but I was dumbstruck. I'm pretty sure my mouth literally dropped open in disbelief.

Then I became offended. Not because of my puritan sensibilities (LOL) or because I was scandalized by the size of his member (I wasn't). I was offended because I'd thought we were both interested in dating, but that picture made me believe he was just looking for a hookup. From my perspective, I had said nothing in our conversation that opened the door for naked photos. Once I got over my initial apoplexy, I was baffled more than anything else. Since I liked this guy, I called him back instead of writing him off.

As soon as he answered the phone, I let loose: "What the hell? Why would you do this? We haven't even kissed, and you're sending me penis pics? That's *not* okay! Normally, I'd assume you're a jerk, and I'd block your number and move on. But I really don't think you meant to be a jerk, so I figured I'd tell you that you crossed a line because I don't want you to do this to somebody else who might get really upset."

Now *he* was baffled.

"What do you mean?" he asked, surprised. "We've been talking about sex for two hours, which is way more personal than a kiss. I thought sending you a picture was hot!"

That's when it smacked me in the head. I was like, *holy shit!*

From his perspective, we'd been experiencing all kinds of intimacy during our phone call—emotional (our past experiences, good and bad), sexual (what we do and don't like), and even romantic (what we might like to do together in the future). This had inspired him to make an exciting, unexpected, sexy, romantic gesture.

Or what he *thought* was an exciting, unexpected, sexy, romantic gesture.

But *to me*, his sending me an unsolicited selfie of his not-so-little soldier was crude and disrespectful—*not* sexy. *Certainly not* romantic.

In hindsight, it's clear to me that my calling him out on it and letting him explain himself led to one of the most enlightening conversations I've ever had. What I learned from him still amazes me; his perspective was so far from anything I'd ever dreamed of.

Do you know why he thought the pic was hot?

Because he didn't feel any shame about his body, even his penis. In fact, to him, it was just a photo of his sexiest body part—the part that proved he was a man. In his mind, sharing this photo was way less intimate than sharing his innermost desires. (As someone who has struggled to love and take pride in her body, I was floored when he said he would have been happy to add that photo to his business card!)

Perspective is everything. Maybe even more so when it comes to sexual etiquette and intimacy.

"If This Is as Good as It Gets, I Need to Get Out"

Romance is encouraged at the beginning of a relationship: romantic weekend getaways, sexy surprises, over-the-top marriage proposals, prom proposals, and now even *homecoming* proposals! Just search "surprise proposal" on YouTube to see the latter for yourself.

But after the wedding day, the big romantic efforts are focused on the next generation: baby showers, gender-reveal parties, birthdays, graduation parties, etc.

It's always struck me as sad that it's only when we—or our relationships—are sick that we pause to consider the idea that our lack of attention to romance might be problematic. We realize with a jolt that we've been phoning in long-stemmed roses at fancy dinners for years, telling ourselves that romance is only window dressing.

Don't get me wrong: I'm not a "roses at fancy dinners" hater! Both roses and fancy dinners *can* be romantic. It depends on the specific people and circumstances involved. Beautiful sunsets and clear, starry nights—these things might be commonplace to some but spectacular to others.

I can't tell you how many couples I meet who assure me that they have a standing weekly date night, celebrate each other's birthdays, and exchange Valentine's Day gifts, but when I ask them to tell me about a recent romantic experience, I get nothing but blank stares and perplexed expressions.

Worse yet is when I see a couple after a big vacation. They'll go on and on, telling me about all the cool things they saw and the exciting things they did. But when I ask them to describe the most romantic part of it, it's like I've asked them to explain general relativity. They'll get a little defensive, repeating themselves by telling me about the Michelin-starred restaurant they went to that required a reservation made months in advance. Although in hindsight, while the food was good, it wasn't as good as they'd expected . . .

Meanwhile, I'll project a dumbfounded expression of my own because what *I* want to hear is more along the lines of what one client shared with me:

"The whole trip was magical, even though we were sick for several days. I got things going by surprising him on the plane with a small gift that got us talking, even touching! By the time we got off the plane, we couldn't wait to get naked in our gorgeous hotel room. We loved the robes so much that we planned to snuggle together in them for an hour a day on our balcony. It was more romantic than our honeymoon. Can you believe that when we went to Le Jules Verne restaurant in the Eiffel Tower, I wore a remote-controlled vibrator that he controlled? The food was good, but we were so excited we skipped dessert in our hurry to get back to the hotel!"

In short, perhaps the simplest way to recognize romantic intimacy is when the circumstances of your situation aren't your main focus.

Rather, the situation serves to create, stimulate, and heighten your feelings overall.

My editor originally wanted to make that last line about good feelings, which opened a fascinating dialogue. The truth is, it isn't always good feelings that create romantic intimacy. Sharing a dark, foggy night with the jitters can be romantic too.[34]

Or take my client who shared with me her experience of going to a haunted house with her boyfriend, who, amid the spooky sounds and masked performers, ran ahead of her in the maze—then leaped out to surprise her a few minutes later. She described it as a little scary, a little exhilarating, and definitely outside the realm of her normal experience . . . a big turn-on!

> Perhaps the simplest way to recognize romantic intimacy is when the circumstances of your situation aren't your main focus. Rather, the situation serves to create, stimulate, and heighten your feelings overall.

Again, when we limit the definitions of intimacy to only uplifting and positive situations, we miss the boat.

I also want to point out that the focus on vacations is not a coincidence. I'm highlighting what I find to be prevalent, and detrimental, among couples—even those who are still happy in their relationship! There's a misguided belief that the particulars of a vacation (or honeymoon or wedding, for that matter) are what will be the measure of "success."

The reality is that couples who are struggling often plan elaborate vacations in hopes of reigniting their love for each other. As if somehow

---

[34] Sometimes going through an emotionally "negative" experience—being scared together on a roller coaster, at a scary movie, or maybe even in a near-miss accident—can bond you. I once went on a whale-watching trip where a woman fractured her leg when she fell right in front of us. Her pain was excruciatingly obvious, impossible to ignore, but when we all got off the boat hours later, strangers were hugging one another.

new settings or magical vistas are powerful enough to transform their relationships while they simply show up. It's like thinking that if you were to visit the Olympic Village, you'd suddenly have the skills to compete in the Games. If only that were so!

What happens instead is the couple will enjoy the trip . . . only to hire a divorce lawyer upon their return home. "The scenery was breathtaking," they'll tell the lawyer, "but when it was just us alone together, it was the same old, same old. Next time, I want to travel with a lover, not just a traveling companion."

Oof.

In case you're wondering, I wasn't the only divorce lawyer whose caseload was heavy with post-vacation filings, especially in August. And we all knew to expect an influx of new cases just after the winter holidays for the same reason.

The moral of the story? It's not so much about where you are, it's about what you do and how you do it.

Recognizing the Romantic Intimacy

I think that, unlike any of the other three intimacies we've talked about, romantic intimacy requires acknowledgment and recognition.

Imagine a couple drinking champagne on a private sunset cruise off the coast of Maui. Doesn't that sound romantic? But wait, let's get a bit closer . . .

Hmmm. Now that we are able to see and hear this couple, it's evident that all is not as idyllic as it first appeared. Sure, they're standing next to each other on the bow of the boat, seemingly watching the sunset, but that's not the whole story. Instead of soaking up the stunning scenery, delighting in the luxurious trappings, while savoring the feeling of being enveloped in a rapturous cloud of romantic bliss . . . they are actually both seething with anger. They're physically tense, strenuously avoiding even an accidental touch, gulping their expensive champagne to stop the angry words that might escape if their mouths weren't otherwise engaged.

It's pretty clear that their refusal to acknowledge or appreciate the romantic ambiance prevents any romantic intimacy.

Creating a passionate, long-lasting love requires that you go out of your way to appreciate romantic opportunities in order to create romantic intimacy.

So what *is* romantic intimacy? It's unique to each of us and our circumstances. You can't just copy someone else's version of it. It's something that has to be cultivated in the moment. It's subject to the subtleties of our mood, expectations, values, desires, and willingness to recognize it.

> Romantic intimacy won't exist unless one allows it to. It is not "one size fits all."

In other words, romantic intimacy won't exist unless one allows it to. It is not "one size fits all."

Maybe your partner loves attending the symphony, in which case, surprising them with tickets might indeed cultivate the perfect conditions for romantic intimacy. But if your partner finds it more romantic to walk through Central Park than sit in a stuffy concert hall, you can save big bucks while still creating romantic intimacy by suggesting a sunset stroll.

Both of these scenarios are okay; they're just different. The key to creating true romance is customizing it for the specific person, which is easier to do when you know what appeals to them. (Note: If you buy the tickets for your symphony fan but your romantic plans are scratched because you're both sick in bed, you might still get credit for creating emotional intimacy since you catered to their particular interest.)

To Be an Adult Is to Be Cool

In the chapter about emotional intimacy, we talked about how young kids aren't shy about letting the whole world know how they feel. But as the years go by, they're discouraged from expressing their emotions via the misguided directive "Behave!"

At the same time, they learn that there is a risk of ridicule, rejection, and/or dismissal if their feelings don't align with those of others around them or meet their expectations. The not-so-subtle lesson exemplified by most adults is this: subdue even your expressions of pleasure and awe in order to protect your image (unless you're drunk, of course!).

I can't tell you how many times others have been embarrassed by my being the first one to clap at the end of a show, getting caught up in belly laughs when someone at the table tells great jokes, or gasping in amazement at David Copperfield's magic. It always strikes me as rather bizarre that while my responses are completely natural, unexaggerated, and appropriate to the situation, I am usually the only adult to wholly succumb to the pleasure of the moment. The others will politely clap once the crowd begins to do so, chuckle discreetly, or nod with a small smile at the most fantastic display.

One of my fellow author friends talks about how rarely people laugh when she's giving a public reading or a presentation, even though her books are funny! But nobody wants to be the first to laugh or do anything that sets them apart from the pack. She says there's nothing she likes less than speaking to a silent room, where she can't tell whether or not people are enjoying themselves.

After a recent reading, she was chatting with a few audience members who were joking around, which gave her the courage to ask why they hadn't been more outwardly enthusiastic during the reading. They were completely surprised by the question. They didn't realize they were holding anything back. (I can't help but doubt that they are so naturally discreet when they stub their toe or trip over their kids' toys at night!)

All this to say, adults can be quite shy when it comes to expressing enjoyment, even romantic pleasure. There's a tendency to contain our feelings until we are sure that those around us "approve." My teenage granddaughter tells everyone who will listen that I cried at the sight of blue whales—on a whale-watching trip, for goodness' sake! I assure you that she does not tell this story because she's impressed with my vulnerability!

This reminds me that while romantic intimacy requires a willingness to allow it, it doesn't mean that one person can prevent the other from experiencing it—though they can make it less likely that the other will do so. On our whale-watching trip, I would have loved it if my granddaughter had been as touched by the sight of these rare, mythical creatures as I was because it would have exponentially increased my pleasure to witness hers.[35]

But her cavalier response didn't have to shut down mine—unless I allowed it to. Instead, I turned my focus back to the utterly miraculous moment at hand as we watched a huge mama whale slowly make her way across our path with her calf by her side. Tears of joy, privilege, gratitude, and awe streamed down my face, just as they are doing now, as I recall that beautiful experience.

I encourage you to start looking at the people around you and try to guess who enjoys romantic intimacy and who doesn't.

I play this game all the time, even going so far as to ask strangers to tell me about their romantic lives. You might be surprised by how many are willing to do so. What I've found is that my guesses are pretty good—though not *always* right, which I love because I love surprises!

---

[35] By the way, here's what National Geographic has to say about blue whales. They are "the largest animals ever known to have lived on Earth. These magnificent marine mammals rule the oceans at up to 100 feet long and upwards of 200 tons. Their tongues alone can weigh as much as an elephant. Their hearts, as much as an automobile." It is estimated that less than 1 percent of people living on Earth will see a whale in their lifetime. Of those, very few will have seen a blue whale, since they are on the endangered species list. Now can you understand why this experience was so incredibly romantic to me? https://www.nationalgeographic. com/animals/mammals/facts/blue-whale.

But generally speaking, it's not hard to recognize the uptight, buttoned-down, anxious, unhappy, tense, terse, stressed-out people who think life is too hard or too short to "waste time" on silly things.

On the other hand, when you see someone who always has a joke to share, even if they aren't funny, someone who laughs freely, ruffles their friend's hair for grins, cries easily, can't resist petting the cute puppy or hugging the lost kid—those are the people who are likely to stop short to delight in the glory of a rainbow, the size of a fish, or the beauty of a symphony. They know that romantic intimacy is the difference between surviving life and *enjoying* life.

> Romantic intimacy is the difference between surviving life and *enjoying* life.

If you want to create romantic intimacy, get personal. Use what you know about your partner to inspire your imagination. Look for ways to surprise them by exploring new areas, seeking adventures, creating excitement, and embracing the unexpected. Maybe even if there's a touch of risk. You don't want to cause real harm, of course, but things that feel a little bit dangerous can be deliciously romantic! Making out in your car, or office, or kitchen when you have family over is a completely safe activity, but it can feel so wonderfully naughty!

When was the last time you were naughty? Who likes to be naughty more, you or your partner? This is a great conversation for the two of you to have because naughty can be such a tantalizing part of romantic intimacy. It gets overlooked, sadly, because popular use of romance is very sappy-centric.

Even if your partner denies having any interest in romance, I want you to dig deeper. I've yet to meet anyone of any gender who doesn't harbor *some* desire for romantic intimacy, even though their version of it might be completely mystifying to anyone else.

Here are a few of the more interesting perspectives I've heard:

- A husband who enjoys taking his wife out to dinner while she wears new shoes, which he purchased for her, because he loves being allowed to kneel at her feet to gently take them off for her when they get home

> Look for ways to surprise them by exploring new areas, seeking adventures, creating excitement, and embracing the unexpected. Maybe even if there's a touch of risk.

- More than a few people who delight in having sex in their boss's office after business hours
- Men who are allowed to wear their female partner's underwear to work or on a date
- An older gentleman whose most fervent desire is for his wife to ride topless in his new, also topless (convertible) car
- A couple who love having sexy fun in the back of a police car
- Men and women who get a charge out of receiving oral pleasure during Zoom meetings

Again, mileage may vary. You can buy chocolate for someone yet not have a single spark of romantic intimacy. Or you can surprise your lover—who has a relentless sweet tooth, especially for Italian chocolate—with last-minute plane tickets to Perugia, Italy, for the international Eurochocolate Festival.

Now *that's* a sweet romance.

Unleash the Unexpected—and Get Extraordinary

Sometimes I describe romantic intimacy as turning the ordinary into extraordinary. You might take a typical event or object that would have virtually no significance to most people and turn it into something extraordinary for your partner, who you know will be into it. It's our perception that shapes what we find romantic.

That's also why I like to stress the unusual and unexpected aspect of romance. Your partner might know you're planning a special date night, for example; it's been marked on their calendar for weeks. But they might *not* be aware of the sexy surprise you've got lined up, which you just know they are going to find so very, very hot. It's something your partner will like but won't expect.

On the other hand, sometimes taking a stab in the dark can hit the bull's-eye.

A while back, I was driving out of town to meet somebody on a first date. When I got there, he still hadn't arrived, so I spent a few minutes sitting at the restaurant, sipping my iced tea and thinking, *Is he going to stand me up?*

Then my phone rang. It was my date calling to explain he'd gotten a flat tire a mile away.

As he apologized, I made a decision. Instead of going home disappointed, I ordered food for two to go. In no time at all, I found his broken-down vehicle on the side of the road. Within minutes, we were enjoying a little picnic on his tailgate.

You know what? It was pretty damn romantic. We waved at all the passing drivers who stared at us as we cracked horrible jokes about my refusal to be stood up. (Humor can absolutely be a part of romantic intimacy, as can fear, anxiety, and the like.)

It wasn't planned. It wasn't sexual. But it was clearly memorable, thanks to the fresh, unexpected energy. It was out of the ordinary. We were both delighted that I'd rolled with the punches so easily. As we lingered on his tailgate, watching a fiery orange sun melt over the Pennsylvania hills, we both agreed it was the most interesting date we'd been on in a long time.

Of course, this can be a tricky line to walk. No matter how well we know our partner, we're still taking a bit of a gamble when we plan something unexpected or surprising. Even when we love and trust our partner, this sense of vulnerability persists. Frankly, the more we care, the more vulnerable we are. That's good for our relationship, but sometimes it feels daunting.

This is why having a good sense of your partner is crucial. The guy who sent me a dick pic thought I would find it romantic. However, he didn't really know me well enough to make that call, so his dick fell short. (Yep, pun totally intended.)

Oops!

I got lucky on that Pennsylvania highway, but romance isn't always that easy.

I'm sure you have seen or experienced a well-intentioned romantic overture gone wrong, right? Someone buys an expensive piece of jewelry that the recipient hates but is now stuck with. Another puts on a piece of lingerie that is way out of her comfort zone, only to be greeted with the shockingly dismayed face of her partner as he asks, "Why are you wearing that?" I surprised my husband with a brand-new Mustang for his fortieth birthday, which I thought would have gotten me not only some lasting romantic intimacy but also the Wife of the Decade award. Nope! A polite "Thank you" was my only reward.

Sure, it sucks to have tried hard only to be summarily dismissed, but it doesn't have to shut you down unless you let it. When these "oops" moments happen, give yourself time to regroup, but then lean in rather than withdrawing. If you can muster the courage to be emotionally intimate with your partner by sharing your feelings about the situation, your relationship will have a much greater chance of success. In a happy relationship, your attempt to rectify the issue will be met with curiosity, kindness, and generosity, which, in turn, will foster greater trust and respect, encouraging more intimacy. That's why intimacy can be an endlessly renewable energy source to keep your love alive.

Opting Out Is Code for Giving Up

Heads up: If you're one of the legions of people who have "opted out" of romance rather than risk a misstep, I strongly suggest you rethink your decision. I've come across untold numbers of people who convince their partners that gifts are foolish, Valentine's Day is nothing more than a commercial fiction, and no one needs candles when they have money for electricity. Suffice it to say that these relationships were far from joyful for both partners.

This brings me to the ugly truth: If either of you steadfastly refuses to learn new ways of creating intimacy, it might be time to consider whether or not your relationship is worth continuing. Don't think that I'm advocating for divorce because I'm not. I'm simply acknowledging that when a partner isn't wholly invested in a relationship, it can be more painful than beneficial to the other. The last thing I want is to encourage anyone to remain unhappy. (Again, been there, done that, and have the divorce decree to prove it.)

Every kind of intimacy is subjective to the individual; romantic intimacy is no exception. Clearly, this can make it a tough nut to crack. Because our culture assigns such specific attributes to the word *romance*—often stereotypically female ones—it can be hard to rewire our brains.

But romance does not belong exclusively to women, nor should it. It has very little to do with Hallmark's pink cards! The original Saint Valentine is rolling over in his grave at what Valentine's Day has become: all the multimillion-dollar marketing firms trying to convince us that romance requires expensive diamonds, flowers, and

> Romantic intimacy is about lingerie. It's about creating feelings that make us quiver and shiver beyond the daily mundane. It's about savoring life fully, embarking on adventures, taking risks, and carving one's own path.

chocolates—hawking the ludicrous idea that every woman has to buy lacy panties to impress her husband on the holiday.

Can lacy panties be romantic? Of course they can! You're talking to a woman who dons lacy bits of lingerie every day! For goodness' sake, I owned a luxury boutique full of elegant lingerie suitable for every type of body and any occasion. But romantic intimacy isn't *about* lingerie. It's about creating feelings that make us quiver and shiver beyond the daily mundane. It's about savoring life fully, embarking on adventures, taking risks, and carving one's own path.

Stop and Smell the Roses—or Whatever You Find Spectacular

The opportunity to enjoy romantic intimacy exists for all of us. It doesn't require big bucks, access to mountaintops, or weeks of planning.

> Romantic intimacy doesn't require another person. You can actually cultivate and celebrate romance with yourself.

If you're about to protest that you'd love to enjoy more romantic intimacy in your life but you can't because you don't have a partner, I'm gonna stop you right there.

Remember my story of being on the beach in Cancún? And my tale of romancing the whales? It may surprise you, but romantic intimacy doesn't require another person. You can actually cultivate and celebrate romance *with yourself.*

It can be as simple as taking yourself on a date. This can be the perfect first date after you've gone through a bad breakup. Think about it: You can treat yourself to exactly what you want, when you want it, and without any concerns for anyone else's preferences. One of my friends dated himself exclusively for six months after a painful divorce. The only reason he started dating other people is because he thought he was spoiling himself too much! (Needless to say, I've learned a lot from Bob; he's a very wise man!)

Romance is the *opposite* of normal.

As an American woman, if I find a beach where I can lay out topless or naked, that can feel very romantic. Why? Because it's unusual. But if I lived in Europe, where many of the beaches are topless or naked, after a while, the romance would probably fade. Nude sunbathing would become just another day at the beach.

Culture often shapes what we perceive as romantic. Sometimes, to find romance, you have to push yourself out of your comfort zone—which might mean challenging the narrative you've lived with.

Another important point worth remembering is this: repetition and easy availability will diminish romance, even in the most loving environment.

Of course, individual people will experience things differently, so something may be romantic to one partner for much longer than it is to the other. Thus, the question is, will you recognize and celebrate your partner's perception of romantic intimacy? Will they do the same for yours? The way I see it, that's the ultimate goal.

Romance Is Like a Slot Machine

One more thing about romantic intimacy: it's fleeting.

But that's okay! I think that's actually a fundamental part of why romantic intimacy is important to keeping love alive.

Not to be overly geeky, but it's human nature to be more responsive to intermittent rewards than constant rewards. That's why slot machines are so compelling. The possibility of a reward keeps us drooling in anticipation; we get a dopamine hit every time. Think of your craving for ice cream versus that of someone

> Occasional bouts of romantic intimacy give us a healthy dose of dopamine that hooks us. It reaffirms our commitment to our relationship, making us want to revisit those feelings again.

who works in an ice cream shop. They're bored with the very *idea* of ice cream. Maybe in their first month on the job, they ate it every single day after their shift. Now they'd be happy to never see an ice cream cone again!

Occasional bouts of romantic intimacy give us a healthy dose of dopamine that hooks us. It reaffirms our commitment to our relationship, making us want to revisit those feelings again.

If romance was constant, it would be "normal," not romantic.

Think of the fireflies that light up the night every summer. Maybe you don't have them where you live, but here in Texas, seeing the first lightning bug of the season is always a delight. If they were around all the time, no one would get excited about them; we'd take them for granted. Those gorgeous insects wouldn't actually be any different, but they'd seem less magical to us.

Let's savor the ephemeral gifts those fireflies give us: a fleeting, extraordinary symphony of sparks across the sky.

Tantalizing Takeaways

- Creating a passionate, long-lasting love requires that you go out of your way to create romantic intimacy.
- Romantic intimacy doesn't require a partner or any sexual intimacy.
- Romance is the opposite of ordinary.

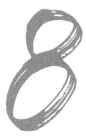

Spiritual Intimacy Ain't About Religion

Spiritual intimacy is the joy of believing, absolutely, that you are in the right place, doing the right thing, with the right person—that you, they, your families, and *the world around you* are better for it.

In this chapter, we'll talk about how to cultivate that sense of confident "rightness" in both yourself and your relationships.

***

When people see the word *spiritual,* they sometimes have a knee-jerk reaction—and not always a good one. They may think this kind of intimacy is about being religious. In reality, spiritual intimacy has nothing to do with religion. Frankly, it's often more problematic for those raised in conservative or religious backgrounds, which can offer us a helpful lens through which to understand it.

> In reality, spiritual intimacy has nothing to do with religion.

I met Rebecca and Sam a few years ago when Hurricane Harvey forced them to cancel their plans for a big vacation to celebrate their twenty-fifth anniversary. They came to my store for some lingerie to make the most of the weekend getaway they had to settle for. (Spoiler alert: while Harvey destroyed their house, it saved their marriage.)

It was impossible not to like them. They were warm, down-to-earth people who were making the best of a bad situation. Even though Rebecca was clearly nervous, she was eager to make their weekend special.

Rebecca and Sam were from small-town Texas; both grew up in very religious families. They fell in love in high school, married soon afterward, and lost their virginity to each other on their honeymoon. They loved God, and they also genuinely loved each other. After twenty-five years of marriage and three kids, they had created the family life they had always wanted.

Sadly, even though things looked perfect, they weren't. The problem was, despite the fact that Rebecca loved Sam as much as she could imagine possible, every time he wanted something more sexually exciting than missionary sex in their bed at night with the lights off, the same thoughts paraded through her head:

He must not respect me.
Good girls don't do that kind of thing.
A godly woman would never say yes to that.

Rebecca couldn't figure out why Sam cared so much about doing different sexy things. She thought he should be satisfied with making gentle love once a week. When pushed, she admitted that she worried he might be a little "perverse" for wanting more.

At the same time, he was feeling like he was stuck between a rock and a hard place. They had everything he wanted in a marriage, and she was everything he wanted in a wife. However, he was so sexually frustrated he'd found himself contemplating divorce—not that he'd mentioned this to Rebecca.

The very thought of divorce made him sick. He didn't want another woman; he just wanted his wife to want him like he wanted her. He wanted to have sexy fun, not BMS.

Until they met me, Rebecca had never even contemplated the idea that sexy stuff was an expression of love or that there was value in it beyond physical release and procreation. She was such a good girl growing up that she'd internalized all the lessons about sex being bad and bringing out the worst in people. She thought of sex as something to put up with rather than a way to make her husband feel loved.

Ironically, working with Rebecca was *my* eureka moment. Up until then, I'd been working with couples on the other four kinds of intimacy, but I hadn't realized that I was taking something for granted: spiritual intimacy.

In Rebecca's heart of hearts, sexual intimacy with her husband detracted from the purity of their love and of her connection to Jesus. She truly believed that it lessened her marriage bond by demeaning her role as an upstanding wife.

I didn't grow up in a religious family, but I understood what Rebecca was struggling with. I think it's really the same thing most girls grow up with: "Sex is something men want from women for their own selfish reasons; women who have sex willingly are 'easy' at best, 'sluts' at worst."

These days, even though spiritual intimacy is listed last in this book, it's the first thing I tackle with all of my clients.

Why?

Because you're never going to truly succeed at creating fulfilling, lasting love if you're wasting energy on inner conflict. Do you think Mr. All-Around Good Guy J.J. Watt could be the NFL superstar he is if he'd been taught that playing football is so shameful, only bad guys play?

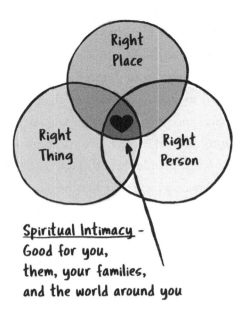

Spiritual Intimacy -
Good for you,
them, your families,
and the world around you

I hate to sound cliché, but until you become really comfortable being completely intimate with yourself—until you are truly open and honest with yourself about your beliefs, values, and deepest sense of what is right, so you can then live your life accordingly—your relationships with others will struggle.

It's not just sexually either. If I think I should keep my house as pristine as those in *Architectural Digest,* but I have kids and I really hate cleaning, what are the chances that I will ever find my home relaxing? Or, for that matter, that my family will?

That's a relatively low-stakes example, but forcing ourselves to do something we don't want to do can have much higher stakes. Consider all the people who might agree to do something but they're not happy about it. Not only do they half-ass it, but they also become resentful. Making this worse is the fact that they're usually upset with themselves for saying yes in the first place! At no time is this more evident than when it comes to sexual intimacy.

Spiritual intimacy starts internally when the way you live your life is in alignment with your values, priorities, morals, and ethics. When you are self-aligned, you'll be ready to find others with whom you can be happy living as your wholehearted, authentic self.

This means the following:

If you are feeling guilty, it is hard to have spiritual intimacy.

If you are feeling shame, it is hard to have spiritual intimacy.

> Until you become really comfortable being completely intimate with yourself—until you are truly open and honest with yourself about your beliefs, values, and deepest sense of what is right, so you can then live your life accordingly—your relationships with others will struggle.

If you are feeling that what you are doing is somehow *not right* or *not good*—however you choose to define rightness or goodness—then it is next to impossible to have spiritual intimacy, no matter how many other kinds of intimacy you may experience.

Spiritual intimacy is our deepest sense of rightness.

In her book *Braving the Wilderness*, Brené Brown put it this way:

> True belonging is the spiritual practice of believing in and belonging to yourself so deeply that you can share your most authentic self with the world and find sacredness in both being a part of something and standing alone in the wilderness. True belonging doesn't require you to change who you are; it requires you to be who you are.[36]

---

[36] Brené Brown, *Braving the Wilderness: The Quest for True Belonging and the Courage to Stand Alone* (Random House: 2017). https://www.amazon.com/Braving-Wilderness-Quest-Belonging-Courage/dp/0812995848.

Right, Good, and Whole: Learning a New Way

When you experience spiritual intimacy, you'll breathe easier. You'll be fully present because it will feel good. You'll feel lighter, enjoy more things, and take pride in all that you do.

If you are a person of faith, it might feel as if you've been blessed by a divine power. If you aren't religious, you might feel you've been blessed by the universe. Or perhaps you'll experience a sense that the moon and stars have aligned, bathing you in radiant warmth.

The ways we experience spiritual intimacy may vary, but it's important to each of us, even those who live their lives outside the law. I know it seems slightly absurd, but even mobsters have a unique code of conduct. (Remember the countless *Sopranos* episodes where the world watched characters struggling to find their own sense of spiritual intimacy despite their outwardly gangster bravado?)

Let's go back to Sam and Rebecca. Even though they had a strong marriage, Rebecca still couldn't let herself enjoy sexual intimacy. All she'd ever heard about sex was that it was dangerous, shameful, wrong, and forbidden. No one had ever thought to tell her when she got married that it was delightful, meaningful, loving, and important. Nor did they point out that there are lots of fantastically exciting ways to enjoy loving her husband. Being the good girl that she was raised to be, Rebecca had never even thought to question her beliefs about sex before she and I started talking.

Rebecca is far from unique in this regard. When we're accustomed to something, it may never occur to us that there is any other way.

When my kids were young, we lived in France for a year. We were shocked to learn that most schools ended at noon on Wednesdays so the kids could play sports. We thought it was the weirdest thing. It had never even occurred to us when we lived in the United States that this was an option. For us, school was five days a week, from 8:00 a.m. to

3:00 p.m. or thereabouts, unless it was a holiday. We assumed—mistakenly—that was the way the world worked because we'd never heard of anything else. Only when we moved to France did we learn a new way.

You can learn a new way too.

Romeo and Juliet: A Spirited (But Not Spiritually Intimate) Love Story

One of the most well-known examples of spiritual intimacy gone wrong is the story of Romeo and Juliet.

High school teachers love to teach this tale—maybe because they know this intense, violent, sexy love story is the best opportunity they've got to convince their students that Shakespeare is cool. Which he was. He never shied away from an emotion or consequence. He delighted in every aspect of the human condition, regaling us with stories that we couldn't help but identify with. In particular, this tale of innocent, ill-fated love has captured the popular imagination for hundreds of years.

Personally, I think it's because he intuitively tapped into an almost universal struggle: how to attain spiritual intimacy.

Romeo and Juliet experience tantalizing physical intimacy. Even in the famous balcony scene, with a whole floor between them, that cool night air is charged with electricity. Before that, they've got that whole thing about touching hands—"palm to palm is holy palmers' kiss." Those crazy kids were hip to the sensual power of handholding long before I was writing about it!

R&J immediately make themselves vulnerable to each other, trading secrets and confidences, sharing emotional intimacy of the highest order. Does Romeo gush about Rosaline, his former crush, on their first date? Not in the text, anyway.

Their whirlwind affair is fraught with romantic intimacy—illicit trysts, a midnight marriage by the friar, even a wild fantasy of escaping Verona to start a new life. Remember, romance means unexpected, surprising, extraordinary, and maybe even a little bit dangerous. R&J's love story has all of that and more.

And—*oh là là*—don't even get me started on the sexual intimacy! Whether your cup of tea is Zeffirelli's 1968 *Romeo and Juliet* or Spielberg's modern-day adaptation, the 2021 *West Side Story*, let's just say you wouldn't be the first to get hot and bothered by R&J's spicy love scene, nor will you be the last.

In case you haven't noticed, there's one glaring absence, one kind of intimacy Romeo and Juliet did *not* have: spiritual intimacy.

Because let me tell you, the world R&J inhabit is rife with strife and bloodshed. The Montagues (Romeo's family) and the Capulets (Juliet's family) hate each other. They are locked in an intense, bloody ongoing family feud.

When Romeo and Juliet fall in love in the midst of this, they know that what they are doing is hurting their families. And this is quite literally, in fact: Juliet's cousin, Tybalt, murders Romeo's best friend, which, of course, leads Romeo to murder Tybalt in a frenzy of revenge.

No one's saying the Montagues and Capulets are being reasonable. They're *not!* But suffice it to say, all that violence and betrayal makes spiritual intimacy nonexistent. Neither Juliet nor Romeo can say, "This is good! This is right! Our families are gonna *love* this."

Shakespeare hit the nail on the head. Huge, passionate, all-consuming love still isn't enough to guarantee a healthy, happy, lasting relationship. If these star-crossed, starry-eyed lovers were doomed by a lack of spiritual intimacy, do any of the rest of us stand a chance?

Feeling Good versus Feeling Guilty

Guilt is the #1 killer of spiritual intimacy.

I don't know why so many of us are so attached to guilt, but it's hard to shake, especially in the realm of romantic relationships. People feel guilty for all sorts of reasons, some rational, some not. Frequently, guilt is associated with fear, such as in the case of a husband with erectile dysfunction who's afraid of "failing," so he avoids sexual intimacy by claiming that he doesn't find his wife attractive anymore, which makes him feel (justifiably, perhaps) like a jerk. Then there's the woman who fell in love with her best friend's ex-husband and now can't figure out why she feels sick at the idea of moving in with him. I could go on for pages, but frankly, I get so depressed by all the unnecessary sorrow that I have to stop.

However, we still need to talk about the most common cause of guilt: affairs.

"If our relationship started when we were both married to other people," a person might ask, "does that mean we destroyed any chance we have at spiritual intimacy?"

Short answer: probably.

"Even if we didn't mean to fall in love? Even if we are blissfully happy together and truly believe we are soulmates, destined to be together forever?"

Again, even the most incredible happiness tinged with guilt results in a deficiency of spiritual intimacy.

If guilt, remorse, and a sense of wrongness are part of your relationship, it's going to be impossible to enjoy spiritual intimacy.

This is the type of nuance that doesn't always get addressed. But it can be the difference between love burning out or love that lasts.

So here's the kicker: to experience spiritual intimacy, you're going to have to excise the guilt, remorse, and sense of wrongness from your relationship.

That's straightforward, right?

As for the execution, that can be a little more complicated, but I can tell you a great place to

> If guilt, remorse, and a sense of wrongness are part of your relationship, it's going to be impossible to enjoy spiritual intimacy.

start. Face your feelings instead of hiding from them. Acknowledge any mistakes you've made and accept responsibility for them. Forgive yourself. Make amends to those you may have harmed.

I'm not the first one to come up with this, of course. Alcoholics Anonymous's *Big Book* has been helping alcoholics achieve spiritual intimacy with this step for almost one hundred years. [37]

Between Home and a Happy Spot

One place I often see a heartbreaking lack of spiritual intimacy is among aging couples. As people get older, their partners might transition to senior centers, nursing homes, or at the most difficult end of the spectrum: memory-care units as they struggle with Alzheimer's disease or dementia. There's a growing number of relatively healthy spouses who love and are devoted to a partner who has been physically, emotionally, or mentally incapacitated for years or even decades.

The trouble for these "surviving" spouses is not of disregard but of love. Being faithful to their incapacitated spouse is important to the healthier partner, but at the same time, they have their own needs that simply aren't getting met. It's all too common for these devoted care-taking spouses to find themselves drawn to somebody who's equally committed to their own ailing partner. They bond over the pain of watching their beloveds suffer. Before long, their emotional intimacy begets a desire for more. I'm sure almost all of us would agree that it's understandable, but when the pleasure of connection collides with guilt, it can be overwhelming to an already overburdened spirit.

This is why I strongly advocate for a couple to address the possibility of a lengthy decline long before they reach their golden years.

---

[37] *Alcoholics Anonymous: The Story of How More Than One Hundred Men Have Recovered from Alcoholism*, 4th ed. (New York: Alcoholics Anonymous World Services, Inc., 2002).

The process should be no different than that of putting together the other planning documents regularly recommended by lawyers, but this would be a moral release rather than a legal one. It should serve as notice to children, family, and even friends that, upon specified circumstances, the marriage may continue but in an "open" fashion. In other words, each spouse is explicitly granted permission to have other relationships that include as many intimacies as they choose. (The common term to describe such a relationship is *ethical non-monogamy*.) Did you notice that I said *each* spouse? That wasn't an error. It's a recognition that senior living facilities are actual hot spots for new love. Just because an Alzheimer's patient can't remember their spouse doesn't mean they don't crave all kinds of intimacy. Denying them consensual pleasure seems cruel to me.

Spiritual intimacy is best when it's experienced by both partners. That means the feeling of rightness flows freely from both directions. If your partner is 100 percent confident that everything is good, but you are not, then you're not going to share spiritual intimacy. A few common examples of this include a husband who's lost his job and doesn't feel "man" enough to be with his successful wife, no matter how much she adores him; a wife consumed with guilt for leaving their kids alone while she and hubby make love in their room with the door locked; or a worried spouse afraid that their guests in the next room will hear their bed squeak.

> Spiritual intimacy is best when it's experienced by both partners. That means the feeling of rightness flows freely from both directions.

In the short term, situations like these may not doom your relationship. They're certainly no Romeo and Juliet, but they certainly deserve your attention and efforts to resolve them sooner rather than later.

Getting Unstuck Can Be Fun!

This brings us back to Rebecca and Sam. You'll never guess how they finally began having hot, juicy, passionate, loving sexy fun . . .

Bible study.

Seriously.

Okay, well, I'm pretty sure *I* helped too, but still!

It was clear that Rebecca needed to live in a manner that was consistent with her faith, but she had to get clarity about what her "faith" actually was. She realized that she wanted to live her life in accordance with Jesus's teachings, but there were serious inconsistencies in what she had been taught versus what she believed. Thus, it was time to throw everything out so she could start from scratch. For those of you struggling to reconcile your faith and your love, I highly recommend the book *God and Sex: What the Bible Really Says*. It provides a thorough, nonjudgmental, nondenominational review of the Old Testament, the New Testament, and the Scriptures.[38] It was recommended to me by a Methodist minister, and I'm forever grateful. I found it to be engaging, compelling, and very eye-opening![39] Written by a Harvard theologian, it's my kind of Bible study.

You'll be happy to learn that, seven years later, Rebecca and Sam are more happily married than ever before. Their lives are full of joy, respect, and an abundance of loving laughter. Rebecca put it brilliantly: "I've always loved him, but now, I love loving him!"

---

[38] Here's a teaser from when Ruth (with coaching from her mother-in-law, Naomi) uncovers Boaz's feet: "And it shall be, when he lieth down, that thou shalt mark the place where he shall lie, and thou shalt go in, and uncover his feet, and lay thee down; and he will tell thee what thou shalt do." I'm gonna let you guess what the word *feet* is a euphemism for . . . https://www.amazon.com/God-Sex-What-Bible-Really/dp/0446545260.

[39] I asked the minister (on air) whether he thought Jesus was a virgin when he died—and he declined (politely) to answer!

Not to be outdone, Sam loves to brag that every Sunday, Rebecca gives thanks to Jesus for the privilege of loving him *frequently*.[40]

Now, maybe you think it's weird that a "nice Jewish girl" like me is so excited about Jesus. But as far as I'm concerned, Jesus is synonymous with love—so of course I'm a big fan! In fact, one of my other favorite client expressions came from a wife of thirty-six years who bragged, "The more I love my husband, the more we please each other, the closer to Jesus I feel."

Can I get an *amen?*

Oh, you might also be interested to know that Rebecca went on to model for my shop in lingerie that covered at least as much as a bikini. She shared some of her photos on social media . . . only to be Jesus-shamed. It was awful. But she didn't let it stop her from living her life exactly how she wanted to. She publicly declared her body a gift from God; she was proud to brag about using it to love her hubby. She refused to be embarrassed any longer by anything God had given her.

I like to think that a big part of why I'm able to help so many people with their deeply personal, complicated relationship issues is my ability to think completely outside the box.

Speaking of which, wanna know how going to a swinger's club saved my clients' marriage?

Getting into the Swing of Things

That's right: I sent an older, conservative couple to a swinger's club to resolve their spiritual intimacy problems. And it worked so well that they are now happy regulars.

Why did I do that? Because after almost forty years of marriage, Joe and Julie still had a great relationship overall. They had a lot of love for

---

[40] Insert all the eggplant emojis your heart desires.

each other, but their sexy passion had reached a plateau that frustrated them both.

They had drawers full of sexy props and a closet stuffed with erotic attire, but it wasn't enough. They wanted something new, something exciting. They racked their brains but came up with nothing workable. They admitted to considering threesomes, but they were firmly committed to maintaining their monogamy.

It didn't take long for them to agree to what I thought was a perfect option: dress to impress . . . for a trip to the local swingers club. There, they could meet and mingle with as many people as they wanted to, soak up all the sexy vibes, and flirt wildly before using the experience to stimulate sexy intimacy between (only!) themselves. Plus, they'd have the option of getting busy at the club, in the car, on the way home, or even at a hotel.

This worked so well for them, aligning completely with their sense of "good," that it created even more appreciation, trust, and pleasure between them. It was like winning the intimacy lottery; each date night won big on all five fronts—emotional, physical, sexual, romantic, and spiritual intimacy!

I can't help but laugh as I'm writing this. I know my deceased mother is rolling her eyes, thinking, *Only my crazy daughter would think to send a straitlaced, gray-haired couple to a swingers club!* But I have no regrets, and more importantly, neither do Joe and Julie.

That's not to say they weren't incredibly nervous the first time they went. That was natural; they were, after all, trying to relearn some fundamental ideas they'd clung to their whole life. Whereas my family had to learn that school could let out early on Wednesdays, Joe and Julie had to come to terms with some truly radical new concepts: that sexy stuff doesn't have to be *utterly* private and being around others who don't live within the bounds of monogamy isn't bad or sinful. It's just totally different—and a big turn-on!

So they worked through it. Their marriage became stronger than ever as they found themselves enjoying loads of guilt-free, wholehearted sexy fun along the way.

Don't you just love a good love story?

Here's another unique one for you. Kendra and Maurice had been happily married in an ethically non-monogamous relationship (they'd mutually agreed it was okay to enjoy sexy fun with others) for eight years, but they had a unique "sticking point." Kendra hated giving oral sex. In keeping with my advice that no one should do something they can't do wholeheartedly, Kendra refused to go down on Maurice even though she knew how much he wanted it. What's interesting is that Kendra didn't think this should be a big deal since they were active in the local swingers community where there were plenty of women who were happy to provide Maurice with oral pleasure.

However, to her utter confusion, no matter how many other women offered to pleasure him, Maurice still wanted it from Kendra. This didn't make sense to her because she thought a blow job was just a means to a "lazy man's orgasm." She had no idea the sexual intimacy she and Maurice shared meant much more to him than the sex he had with others. When he was with her—even though he didn't know how to describe it until working with me—it was emotional, physical, sexual, romantic, and, yes, *spiritual intimacy*, all rolled up together in a delicious love wrap. He wanted her whole body to love his whole body. Her unwillingness to do so was more than a lack of sexual intimacy; it felt like a major rejection of his importance to her (negative emotional intimacy because she knew how much he wanted it), while also making him doubt his physical attractiveness (negative physical intimacy).

Upon hearing it put this way, Kendra cried. She couldn't believe that something she considered trivial meant so much to the man she loved. She hated that she'd unwittingly been hurting him for so many years. Determined to make amends as quickly as possible, she signed up for my

How to Blow His Mind While Loving His Body video class. Wow. What a difference a little enlightenment and education made! Kendra told me the class "blew the lid off everything" she'd thought she knew. Her new knowledge, combined with the confidence she gained, completely transformed their marriage. Going down on Maurice became one of Kendra's favorite parts of their sexual intimacy. It flooded her with feelings she described as "ecstatic harmony." She is now free to love him wholly with her head, heart, spirit, and body—which feels exactly right. And needless to say, Maurice feels like he hit the marriage jackpot!

If you're at all like I was ten years ago, you might be a bit shocked to think that Bible study, lingerie modeling, swingers clubs, and oral sex can all be the secret sauce for a happy, healthy marriage. I get it; it still surprises me when I see "loving miracles" happen. All I can tell you is different strokes making different folks happy makes life wonderfully interesting!

Learning to Swim

Here's a sweet story about getting unstuck. When my daughter was learning to swim, she would do one stroke with one arm while clinging to the lane divider with the other.

People do the same thing with love. Sometimes we cling to the past because we're so scared of drowning in a new relationship. Maybe we're clinging to a set of religious or moral beliefs we inherited from someone else. Or maybe we've learned being vulnerable leads to harm.

Whatever your fear is, you might not be able to imagine anything working out differently. You hold on to it because you think it protects you, keeps you safe. That's only natural, especially if you've been hurt in the past. In truth, it *does* protect you, in a way. Continuing our pool analogy, if you've just had a muscle cramp and need to relax for a few moments to recover, holding that lane divider is the perfect way to do so. On the other hand, if that muscle spasm was hours ago and you're still holding on because you're terrified you'll have another one, it's probably time to move on.

Before you let go, you should assess the situation with open curiosity, assuage your fears kindly, give your body what it needs, and invite your mind to work through the options. Decide whether to seek help or proceed alone. These are the steps that will assure you that you are making the right choice for your best possible future.

Spiritual intimacy is what gives you the courage to let go and move forward.

If you are in a relationship that you want to invest in more deeply, you're going to have to let go of the lane divider.

> If you are in a relationship that you want to invest in more deeply, you're going to have to let go of the lane divider.

Tantalizing Takeaways

- Spiritual intimacy is the joy of believing, absolutely, that you are in the right place, doing the right thing, with the right person—that you, they, your families, and *the world around you* are better for it.
- Blame, shame, guilt, and obligation are the most common killers of spiritual intimacy.
- A lack of spiritual intimacy is likely to significantly detract from your level of fulfillment with the other kinds of intimacy.

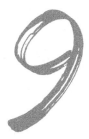

The Tango of the Intimacies

As you now understand, the intimacies are the substance of love, adding practical value to life in ways that a mere emotion cannot. Clearly, each of the five intimacies can stand alone, but ideally, all the intimacies are interwoven, braided together to make your relationship as strong as it can possibly be. While each thread—each intimacy—is vital, contributing something uniquely significant, when combined, the sum is significantly greater than the parts.

If you prefer a food metaphor, each intimacy has its own nutritional value that contributes to the overall health of your relationship, making it stronger to become a more vital part of your life. While you could achieve a balanced diet by eating one food group at a time, your pleasure is magnified when you enjoy them in concert as a meal.

> Remember that just like no amount of sugar will satisfy your body's need for protein, an abundance of one kind of intimacy will not make up for the lack of another over the long term.

Remember that just like no amount of sugar will satisfy your body's need for protein, an abundance of one kind of intimacy will not make up for the lack of another over the long term.

This brings us to the most important part of this book: How do you use what you've learned to actually change your life?

Don't be nervous! I promise it's going to be fun. The journey will also be illuminating, insightful, and—yes—maybe a little uncomfortable. But on the other side of that discomfort are great big gobs of joy, laughter, and delight. Think of it as training for a marathon of love!

As every good chef knows, there are some flavor combinations that simply don't work well and others that make our tongue dance with delight. In this chapter, we'll look at the ways the different intimacies interact in romantic relationships, in both healthy and unhealthy ways. We'll talk about the places where there's often a disconnect between intimacies. I'll share some of the most common issues faced by my clients over the years in the hope that their experience will make yours easier.

When it comes to incorporating the five intimacies into your relationship, think of it as learning to dance with your partner. When you master the five intimacies, things will flow so easily it'll feel like your feet are gliding seamlessly over the dance floor. If you stumble, your partner will catch you and help you find your rhythm again—and vice versa. No matter what happens, you'll share it all together: having fun, holding each other close, and moving together to create something beautiful.

On that note, I want to introduce you to Amy and Todd.

Mastering the Make-Out Session

When I met Amy, she was a dynamic woman in her early forties, married to her professed dream guy. Even though she gushed about how much she loved him because he was so amazing, she also admitted that their sex life was practically nonexistent. Sure, they still found each other attractive, but between demanding jobs, three kids, and their active social lives, sex had been relegated to an afterthought.

While the lack of sex wasn't a huge concern for Amy because not one of her married friends was doing any better, what bothered her was that she no longer cared when their date nights needed to be canceled. In fact, when prodded, she admitted she was even a bit relieved. Spending time alone with Todd used to be one of her favorite ways to enjoy an evening; now, she was thrilled to crawl into bed alone with a book. Even though they lived together and everything *looked* the same, there was a marked change in the way she and Todd acted toward each other. Not only was there no PDA, but there also was some subtle avoidance of physical interaction. They didn't talk about it, but she realized they both avoided touching or hugging the other, awkwardly backing away to let the other pass without the "accidental" rubs they used to enjoy at every opportunity.

When questioned about this, Amy explained that Todd wanted more sexy fun, but since *she* didn't, she avoided physical connection so he wouldn't take it as an invitation for sexy fun. She didn't want him to accuse her of leading him on. Worse yet, she didn't want to do anything to encourage him to think about their lack of sexual intimacy.

Meanwhile, Todd felt like Amy didn't find him attractive anymore because every time he touched her, she pulled away. Of course, even if he just wanted a hug, she was probably telling herself something along the lines of, *Oh great, all he wants is sex.*

They'd been locked in that pattern for so long that physical touch in their relationship had started to have a negative association for both of them.

Argh! I see this dynamic so often, I'd say it's practically an epidemic. I guess the upside, though, is that the antidote is pleasure.

Toward that, I asked Amy to tell me what she missed doing with Todd, what *used to* make her excited at the thought of spending time with Todd.

"Todd and I used to make out like crazy," Amy replied wistfully. "I *loved* the way he kissed. We would make out for hours."

They clearly had sexual chemistry. But for Amy, there was also emotional intimacy in that kind of kissing.

When I asked how long it had been since they'd made out, Amy was shocked to realize it had been years. Since sexual intimacy had become a point of contention, they'd sacrificed all physical intimacy, including things they both really enjoyed. So it shouldn't be a surprise to you that they weren't enjoying much of any of the remaining intimacies either. They were so hopelessly knotted up that neither Amy nor Todd had a clue how to untangle what was becoming an ugly hairball.

So I gave them a rule as well as an assignment: I said, "No sex for two weeks, but make out as often as you want."

Boy, did that unleash unexpected passion!

The two of them spent the time making out. And making out. And making out some more. The next time she came to see me, her eyes were sparkling as she grinned like the Cheshire cat, saying, "Sorry, Beth. We broke your rules! Repeatedly. We tried to just make out, but it felt so good we couldn't *not* have sex. We'd try again the next day, but before we knew it, we were naked on the couch again! It's a good thing our kids are sound sleepers!"

Isn't that awesome? Don't you want what they've got?

All it took was a simple mental switch from focusing on what was lacking (goal-oriented sexual activity) to committing to *having fun*. They could make out for a minute or for hours; there would be no presumed beginning, middle, or end. When they were free to focus only on what was pleasurable for both of them, for only as long as it was pleasurable, loving each other became joyful again.

Yes, amping up their physical intimacy resulted in reinvigorating their sexual intimacy as well—but that was a perk, not the end goal. It's also important to remember that I chose "making out" as the homework assignment because Amy had specifically identified it as something they had both really enjoyed in the past. If she had said they liked holding hands while skipping through the park, I would have "prescribed" that. The point is we enter relationships because they're *fun* and they feel good; if they stop being pleasurable, we have little incentive to continue them.

I don't know what your relationship is like, but simple adjustments, such as the one I described above, often lead to big improvements, in part because of the human body's chemistry. When Amy and Todd made out, they both got a natural high from what I affectionately call *happy hormones*. Their make-out sessions stimulated oxytocin, dubbed the "love hormone."[41] And as if that weren't enough, they also got a big dose of dopamine, nicknamed the "feel-good hormone."[42] In other words, if you tune in to your body, you'll notice it responds to pleasurable touch with extraordinary delight!

> The point is we enter relationships because they're fun and they feel good; if they stop being pleasurable, we have little incentive to continue them.

Amy had wasted so much time being annoyed that Todd wanted sexual intimacy that she completely forgot that her body wanted pleasure too!

Voilà! We call that two birds with one sexy kiss.

Emotions and Sex: Not Always a Love Story

Another disconnect I see among my clients is when a couple has regular sexual intimacy—but zero emotional intimacy. That often surprises people. "If a couple is having sex," they ask, "how can they *not* be connecting emotionally?"

---

[41] Stephanie Watson, "Oxytocin: The Love Hormone" (Harvard Health Publishing, July 20, 2021), https://www.health.harvard.edu/mind-and-mood/oxytocin-the-love-hormone.

[42] "Dopamine: What It Is, Function & Symptoms," Cleveland Clinic, https://my.clevelandclinic.org/health/articles/22581-dopamine.

Believe it or not, you could be having sexy fun with your partner three times a day—sexy fun you very much enjoy—and still not share any significant emotional intimacy.

You could also be having boring, uninspired, by-the-book sex that is *not* fun—which is way more common—yet have lots of emotional intimacy.

I see it all the time: couples with a huge disconnect between their emotional and sexual intimacy levels.

"But, Beth," you might say, "I love having sex with my partner. It's fantastic! I have multiple orgasms every time we hook up."

To this, I'd reply, "Terrific! I wish you all the orgasms you could ever want. But even at the height of the best, most mind-blowing orgasm of your life, with a partner you love dearly, satisfying emotional intimacy isn't a given."

Ironically, I know lots of people who have what they consider their best sexy fun with partners with whom they have no emotional intimacy nor desire for it.

If you think about it, the lack of emotional intimacy offers some freedom. We aren't invested in what that person thinks or needs. We don't have to share anything significant about ourselves. And it's easy to walk away quickly if things become unpleasant in any way. There are lots of people who enjoy sex without emotional entanglements because it's easy to compartmentalize.

The problem is when this is within the framework of a marriage or another kind of committed relationship, it's likely that at least one partner is under the mistaken impression that regular sexual intimacy alone will ensure a happy relationship or make up for the lack of other intimacies. This is no less likely if a relationship has healthy emotional intimacy but little other intimacy.

As a divorce lawyer, I had a roster of clients who, despite having little to no sexual intimacy with their spouse, thought their marriage was strong because they were "best friends" (emotional intimacy) . . . right up until they were completely shocked by a request for divorce along with a confession of a long-term affair. (Forgive me for being a Negative Nancy for a moment, but I have a pearl of wisdom for those of you who've been in a sexless marriage so long you're convinced your partner doesn't have any sexual desires anymore. Based on my experiences over three decades on both sides of the fence, I'd say there's a very good chance that the reason your marriage has lasted so long is because your partner is getting their sexual intimacy needs met elsewhere. I know that sounds harsh, but I've seen it far too often to discount it.)

There are also way too many relationships caught up in a cycle of doom because one partner is demanding one kind of intimacy and is unwilling to prioritize anything else until they're "satisfied"—which is usually an impossibility.

I'm embarrassed to admit this, but . . .

That was me too.

It Takes Two to Tango

In my marriage, I had BMS two to three times a week on average for twenty-three years, but I never had any meaningful emotional intimacy.

Outside our bed, we had virtually no other real, deliberate physical intimacy. I mean, we lived together, sharing the same bed, but if it wasn't sexual, we rarely touched.

Obviously, that was a completely dysfunctional relationship. It's painful for me to see that so clearly now, yet while I was in it, I couldn't figure out what the problem was or how to fix it.

My husband and I were caught up in an endlessly destructive cycle of my starving for an emotional connection that I couldn't describe while, at the same time, he constantly craved more sex to fill a void he couldn't identify. Neither of us realized that no amount of sexual intimacy was ever going to satisfy our innate, undeniable, totally human need for emotional intimacy.

What's really crazy to me as I now look back is that neither of us had *ever* experienced much positive emotional intimacy. You might think—the way we clearly did—that we wouldn't miss what we didn't know. But it's so clear in hindsight that, subconsciously, something deep within both of us hungered for that which we didn't know.

I cringe when I think about all the years of him saying, "I want more sex. I'm miserable because we don't have enough sex. I'd be happy if . . ." and me, lying next to him after sex, feeling lonely and sad, and beating myself up for wanting something I couldn't name instead of being happy with what I had.

Of course, over the years since then, I've also seen the flip side of this: people who refuse to engage in sexual intimacy until their emotional intimacy needs are met. Yet their subconscious issues prevent their hearts from ever registering as "full," so they never "have to" be sexually intimate.[43]

If you're not investing in and being fueled by all 5 Kinds of Intimacy, your relationship is operating at a deficit. It may continue, but it will do so in dysfunction.

> If you're not investing in and being fueled by all 5 Kinds of Intimacy, your relationship is operating at a deficit. It may continue, but it will do so in dysfunction.

Remember our braid metaphor? When all five intimacies are a part of that braid, it increases the flexibility and strength of a relationship. This means that any weakening of one intimacy can be tolerated because of the strength of the others, allowing the couple time to make repairs before serious damage is done.

---

[43] Whenever you see a couple frantically trying to get "more, more, more" of any kind of intimacy, it's a safe bet there are some codependency issues.

Undoubtedly, you'll experience dips in one kind of intimacy or another over the course of your relationship. Circumstances change, health issues occur, and family crises are almost inevitable over a lifetime. Job changes, childbirth, mental health issues, loss, and grief all have serious effects on how much energy we have to devote to our relationship and how much effort we can invest in creating intimacy.

This is why you need to become adept at creating each kind of intimacy when things are good. You need to be prepared for rough times. You have to understand that, yeah, you're taking these one or two kinds of intimacy off the table, but you'll find workarounds until you get back to them.

The lulls in each intimacy should be temporary, not allowed to linger longer than absolutely necessary. This is important because it will help ensure that neither partner becomes resentful during this period. You don't want to be in a situation in which one person is deliberately withholding from the other, saying something along the lines of, "Hey, I'm not getting sex, so I'm not even going to bother talking to you. I'm not going to call you or check in with you." That's obviously not a recipe for success!

But if you're empathetic, supportive, and forthcoming with each other, you'll make it through the hard times. Strong relationships can overcome them—and might even emerge stronger as a result.

What's in It for You?

I gotta say, I feel for you, men.

As we talked about in chapter 5, our culture does not teach men that it's okay to have emotions. In some ways, this has gotten better in recent years; there are certainly more young men who are able to express their feelings.

But there's still plenty of judgment—not to mention shame—directed at men when they are emotionally vulnerable.

If you want to see a grown man squirm, ask him, "What do you feel?" Then don't let him off the hook until he gives you a sincere answer.

I jest, but not much. The sad reality is that most men find it incredibly difficult to delve into their hearts to figure out how they feel, which is why emotional intimacy is so difficult for them. But until they understand what they want and "get" from sexual intimacy, I can't help them achieve it in other ways. (Of course, they "get" orgasm, but they can experience that while alone, so if they prefer sexual intimacy with a partner, there have to be other benefits like excitement, a sense of pride in being wanted, or the ability to give pleasure, physical affection, affirmation of worthiness, joy, a feeling of connection.)

So I routinely pose questions such as these:

"What do you feel while in the midst of sexy stuff? And afterward?"
"Is there a difference to you between making love and having sex?"
"What made the greatest sex you've had so great?"
"What's your favorite part of sexual intimacy?"

Sometimes I have to dig a little to get men to answer these questions sincerely and without their making jokes. Occasionally, they are remarkably open right off the bat, which tells me that they're going to be great at emotional intimacy. No matter how long it takes for me to receive answers, the prevailing responses are along these lines:

"I feel proud."
"I feel desired."
"I feel lucky that she chose me."
"I feel powerful."
"I feel wanted."
"I feel like a man."

Is this what you were expecting?

You can't spend time talking with as many men as I have (with clothes on, I should add!) and not realize that they want love just as much as women do. Sure, they're entranced by orgasmic sexy adventures, but those are just the means by which they hope to attain something more meaningful—passionate, intimately fulfilling love, to be specific.

If we can help them feel all those warm, fuzzy feelings in other ways, then I think everyone wins—the same way women enjoying emotional intimacy by way of sexual intimacy is a win-win. This isn't because we stop emphasizing either one but because we all deserve as many avenues as possible to get what we need and want.

This is why each of us is responsible for identifying what we want from each of the five intimacies. Once we do, we can say to ourselves, "Okay. Are these reasonable expectations? Or am I setting impossible standards so I'll never be satisfied?" If we're good with our desires, we can then start trying to satisfy them through the intimacies.

This approach can be especially transformative for men with erectile dysfunction issues or anything else that makes them feel "less than" in the bedroom. The same goes for women after undergoing a mastectomy or anything that makes *them* feel "less than." It's not just about what you look like; it's how you feel on a deeply personal level, what you think you have to offer a partner.

The truth is that everyone, no matter how uniquely abled they are, has something wonderful to offer a partner. You just have to be open to allowing joyful pleasure in different ways. The easiest way to do so is to start with whatever you know or imagine will feel good. It's super simple but extremely powerful. Make it an adventure, one you can explore with your partner. Try new things; if they don't feel good, don't do them again. If you like them, do them a lot! Don't restrict your definition of pleasure to orgasm. Also, don't assume you need an erection to give pleasure. Just ask your favorite lesbian if that's necessary!

Appreciate What You Have

Most marriages have a lot of physical intimacy (because they live together), but very few couples appreciate or even acknowledge it. Tender moments, such as straightening the other's tie or fastening a necklace, are taken for granted. Opportunities for stolen kisses are overlooked. Meals are rushed or mindlessly consumed in front of the television.

Living together can quickly seem rote rather than intimate, but as any widow will tell you, enjoy even the smallest of things because you'll miss them like crazy when they're gone.

With this in mind, there are endless opportunities to use the physical intimacy you already share as a platform upon which to create more intimacy in other areas. I'm sure you can think of your own ideas, but if you want some more ideas to kick-start your creative juices, here are a few:

- Institute a dinnertime ritual in which each person shares the best and worst parts of their day.
- Before kissing your partner good night, tell them about one of your favorite memories of them or about something you're looking forward to sharing with them in the future.
- Agree to hug for one minute at least twice a day.
- Agree to both sleep naked once a week.
- Offer to wash your partner's back when they shower or bathe.

I think you'll be happily amazed by what a difference you can make in only a couple of minutes a day. You'll also develop more awareness of what works best for each of you, so you'll learn to be more deliberate, cultivating intimacy in ways that truly satisfy. Knowing what you do now about intimacy, it should be fairly easy to make more of the physical intimacy that already exists in your relationship, but I hope you don't stop there.

Have you ever heard about the Hidden Mickeys at Walt Disney World? They're subtle, not meant to be immediately noticed or obvious. The challenge is to be aware enough of your surroundings that you notice these extra little surprises. Each time you do, you get a little zap of dopamine (the "feel-good hormone"), which elevates your Disney experience beyond your expectations. Like the slot machines I mentioned earlier in the book, the chance to "win" by discovering a Hidden Mickey keeps us engaged, excitedly seeking the next one.

Your relationship is like your own personal world of hidden intimacies. There are unmined sources of deep intimacy hidden in almost every relationship, even those that are struggling. As we discussed in the preface, every act of love, regardless of the particular "love language," is a potential source of intimacy waiting for you to substantiate your love.

Once you identify an act of love or another source of potential intimacy based on someone's reaction (positive or negative) to it, the best way to reveal the hidden power is to ask a series of "why" questions to each other. ("Why is this affecting you?" "Why are you afraid to acknowledge the impact this is having on you?" "Why does this make you want to run away?") The reason you need to ask a series of these questions, instead of just one, is because our first, second, and sometimes even third answers are typically superficial. Our emotional truth is usually buried so deep that we have to seriously dig just to get to it.

I know this is hard to understand, so let me give you an example to help explain it.

Scott and Roberta grew up having to fend for themselves from the time they were toddlers because they both had parents who were more consumed with their own needs than those of their children. Their independence is what allowed them to mature into professionally successful adults, but it also hindered their ability to be emotionally intimate despite the love they felt for each other.

Committed to finding the "hidden intimacies" in their relationship, I asked them to think of something the other person had said or done that made them feel good. Roberta's face lit up as she told me she liked that Scott made her favorite buttery corn muffins for her breakfast on Saturday mornings. Even better, he always had them ready for her by the time she'd finished her morning workout. When asked why this was significant to her, she happily described how yummy the muffins were. I admitted they sounded delicious but pointed out that if he loved them as much as she did, she probably wouldn't have ranked that as one of the best parts of her week. I again asked her why it made her feel so good, suggesting that she dig deeper into her feelings for clarity. After a few fits and starts, she realized that finding her favorite breakfast waiting for her made her feel nurtured, special, cared for in a way she had never felt as a child. *Bingo!* Here was a hidden intimacy!

Scott's act of service wasn't hidden—it was an obvious act of service intended to express his love—but the way it affected and created feelings of intimacy for Roberta *was.* She had, of course, thanked him, telling him how much she loved the muffins. What she hadn't revealed, possibly hadn't even noticed herself, was how this simple act filled her heart in a surprisingly wonderful way. When I asked why she hadn't let Scott in on the extent of her pleasure, she honestly didn't know. By using a few more "why" questions, I got us to the bottom of that issue: fear. Sounds weird that there would be any fear related to someone doing something nice for us, right? But it was a perfectly rational response for Roberta, given that throughout her childhood she'd repeatedly learned that even if someone did something for her once, the chances of it happening again, let alone repeatedly, were slim to none. Put simply, it was safer for her to avoid enjoying anything too much because then she'd just be disappointed when it was taken away from her.

The sad irony of this is if Scott doesn't realize it's meaningful to Roberta, he won't prioritize it in the future. Now that he knows it's a big deal to her (feels emotionally intimate), he's thrilled to touch her heart every weekend!

What makes this even more of a win-win is that after a lifetime of feeling unimportant and insignificant, Scott now gets to savor the fact that Roberta is hungry for his attention. Knowing how important he is to her emotional well-being fills him with joyful pride, and it creates emotional intimacy for *him* as well. Everyone wins! Woo-hoo!

But wait, there's more!

Never forget that great intimacy comes with great responsibility. If you don't want to cause further damage to the ones you love, you need to truly accept them for who they are rather than expect them to handle everything rationally. In this instance, Roberta's sensitivity to disappointment *must* be respected. It doesn't matter that she's in her forties; what matters is that her heart is particularly sensitive in this area. Failure to have a plan for the inevitable Saturday morning when this ritual is impossible for one reason or another is begging for trouble. With this in mind, we agreed that when he couldn't make her breakfast, Scott would give her as much advance warning as possible, take care of his own feelings to avoid guilty defensiveness, and then assure her that he would do it again, starting on a specific date. The combination of these things should minimize the chance of Roberta giving in to her fear of rejection, imagining that she's not important enough to him or convincing herself that it will never happen again.

The last item of note is that even though Roberta craved this kind of nurturing intimacy, it wouldn't be surprising for resistance to kick in at some point. Signs of fighting a deepening dependency might appear as her sudden dislike of the muffins, resentment that he "expects" her to be happy every weekend, or suspicion that he's only doing this to make himself look good. I encouraged Scott and Roberta, if or when either of them senses resistance, to create more intentional physical intimacy throughout the week to combat it.

Hidden intimacies can be found in the tiniest of things, whether they're intentional expressions of love, incidental courtesies, or acts of aggression. They can include finding the porch light left on for you, knowing your partner won't leave in the morning without kissing you goodbye, receiving a good night text when traveling, and coming home to a fridge full of healthy food instead of beer. For Scott, finding an open garage door when he came home each day felt like Roberta had hung up a party banner reading, *I'm glad you're here!* If you relinquish expectations about what "should" matter when you start looking for the hidden intimacies in your relationships, I think you'll be amazed to find what *does* matter. With committed intention, you can create positive intimacy from almost anything. Then you can start creating your very own uniquely fulfilling intimacy tango.

Tantalizing Takeaways

- If you're not investing in and being fueled by all 5 Kinds of Intimacy, your relationship is operating at a deficit.
- As you increase your level of one kind of intimacy, it is likely to have a rollover effect, improving other kinds as well.
- Each of us experiences and appreciates each kind of intimacy in different ways. Discovering what works best for your relationship is important and will create more emotional intimacy at the same time!

10

You Asked; I Answered

Afterter my friend read the first draft of this book, she sent me an email.

Um . . . Beth? she wrote. *I've been with my boyfriend for eleven years, and he's wonderful. Our partnership is really strong. But I gotta say, after reading this draft, I'm not sure we do have all five of the intimacies. Now I'm a little worried!*

She was feeling anxious, and I felt for her because this wasn't the first time someone had expressed these kinds of anxieties after I'd shared with them the five kinds of intimacy. I immediately dashed off a reassuring email, then posed a question of my own to my editor:

"What if we answer a handful of questions up front to allay some of the most common worries people have about the five intimacies?"

She loved the idea. So here we are now, in the Ask Me Anything chapter, where I'm going to share a handpicked selection of some of the most common questions I get asked about intimacy.

We'll start with my friend's.

Dear Beth: I've been with my partner for eleven years and we're still truly, deeply, madly in love. But what if there's one kind of intimacy in which I just don't feel quite as connected to my partner as I do in the other four? Does that mean we're doomed?! – *Curious Couple*

Hi Curious Couple!

Not at all! I'd actually say the opposite: it means you've got some exciting new terrain to explore with the person you're madly in love with inside the container of a relationship that already feels safe and supported.

Also, I want to note that there will be times in all our lives when one intimacy is stronger than the others—and sometimes it is completely unrelated to anything you did or didn't do. Let's say your partner gets a job overseas or enlists in the military, and suddenly they're gone for months (or even years) at a time. You simply can't have physical intimacy. That's not your fault. It certainly doesn't mean your relationship is doomed.

> Each kind of intimacy will naturally ebb and flow through the different stages of your life.

So what can you do in the meantime? Look for ways to crank up the romantic or sexual intimacy, even when physical intimacy isn't an option at the moment. Adapt the exercises in Part Two in any ways you want to make them work for your particular situation.

Most importantly, don't panic. Each kind of intimacy will naturally ebb and flow through the different stages of your life. As long as you remain focused on creating intimacy in whatever ways are available to you, you should be good.

***

Dear Beth: What does real emotional intimacy feel like? Is there something wrong with me that I don't know? – *Somebody's Girlfriend*

Hi Somebody's Girlfriend!

First of all, pat yourself on the back for asking this brave question. It means you're already ahead of the game just by *wanting* to know what real emotional intimacy feels like. Most people never even think to ask.

There is nothing wrong with you. In my work with couples, I see *many* people struggle to answer this question. If anything, the majority are like you: They may have a vague, hazy notion of what emotional intimacy is, but when they actually get down to brass tacks, they're stumped. I get this because it's taken me years to clarify it myself. Sadly, it's still hard to explain, but I'll tell you what I tell my clients:

Emotional intimacy is all about connecting with your heart.

Visualize your heart as a small bottle with a flip top. When it's closed, no matter how much love anyone sends you, nothing's going to get in. If you find a way to open it, love can flow in, which will warm you up from the inside out. Once you learn how to open and close your heart, you can close the lid when you're around people to whom you don't want to give access.

How do you know if you've opened your heart? Think back to a moment when you felt love, whether you were receiving or giving it. For me, one of my first memories of love was when a beloved teacher brought me a gift in the hospital when I got my tonsils removed. I was so taken by surprise by the feelings that I cried. One of my clients experienced love for the first time in kindergarten when she held a kitten. Another first experienced love when his older brother picked him for a kickball team. None of us experience love the same way, but it's often associated with a feeling of lightness, an ability to breathe deeply and relax more fully, an inner warmth, and a sense of safety or comfort.

Do you have that moment in mind? Good. In that moment, your heart was open. Otherwise, you wouldn't have been able to feel love. Now, when you try to open your heart, just remember this or another loving moment. If you feel the same feelings you did when it happened, then your heart is open. If you remember but don't feel anything, it's likely closed. If that happens, don't stress; this takes practice. Just close your eyes and try to open your heart again. It'll get easier with practice, I promise.

Hi Curious Couple!
As for emotional intimacy, well, that's what happens when you have access to someone else's open heart or they have access to yours. Or both. With or without love. But *with* is best.

***

Dear Beth: I recently attended one of your intimacy workshops and really enjoyed it. Hearing you talk about the five intimacies made me realize something I'd never fully admitted to myself: I've enjoyed a lot of success in my career, and my personal life looks great from the outside, but I'm realizing it's not nearly as good as it could be.

Lately, I've really been struggling in all my relationships, not just my marriage. I spend a lot of time trying to figure out when things went wrong between my brothers and me and why I never felt close to my parents. What a waste of time, right? All this snooping around in the past! I lost my mom a few years back, and while I definitely miss her, I don't feel like I ever really knew her. Same with my dad, who's still alive.

I worry this pattern will repeat with my own kids—that when I die, they won't have known the real me. I guess, deep down, I'm afraid that, maybe, if my family really did get to know me, they'd realize I'm not actually worth loving. No matter how hard I try, I'm certainly not a perfect parent or a perfect husband, and I was never a perfect son. What is it that I'm missing? And how do I find it? – *Not Perfect Guy*

Hi Not Perfect Guy!

First off, thank you for writing this. You seem like an honest, courageous man, which is what's going to make you not just professionally successful but also personally successful (well-loved, happy, secure, and confident).

Here's what I want you to hear: love doesn't require perfection, nor is it perfect.

I think your willingness to look at all the important relationships in your life is fantastic. It will help you understand yourself better, which will ultimately help you improve your relationship with your kids and others. It's important to see how our family of origin handled the different intimacies; otherwise, we are doomed to unwittingly repeat the same mistakes.

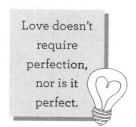

Love doesn't require perfection, nor is it perfect.

None of us should feel guilty for seeing how perfectly imperfect we, our parents, or our children are. If we're unwilling to do so, we can never fully appreciate emotional intimacy with them. And knowing someone shouldn't decrease the love we feel for them; it should increase it. If the *Mona Lisa* teaches us anything, it's that imperfection is captivating. If you doubt this, look at your children. I'm sure they're wonderful; I'm also sure they're imperfect. Could you love them more? I doubt it.

I hope you'll learn to welcome the experience of emotional intimacy and that, in doing so, you'll find yourself extending as much grace to yourself as you do to others around you. If your family is willing to learn with you, that would be great, but it's not necessary. Even if you never talk to them about the work you're doing to cultivate intimacy, the way you interact with them will change things regardless.

I hope this helps you feel okay about "snooping around" in the past. After all, isn't it yours?

***

Dear Beth: When we do the State of Your Union assessment, if we score really low in a certain intimacy, should we drop everything else and focus only on that? I mean, if you were our relationship coach, would you try to fix that kind of intimacy first? – *Nervous Test Taker*

Hi Nervous Test Taker!

Actually, no. Since the lowest score is typically the hardest and most discouraging for people, I suggest you start with whatever is working well and feels easy to you. By doing so, you'll build up confidence in yourself as well as your relationship, which will give you the motivation needed to tackle the more difficult aspects. I'm a firm believer that pleasurable positive reinforcement brings out the best in all of us.

***

Dear Beth: I have a question about romantic intimacy. Can this kind of intimacy occur between two people when one of them isn't even aware of it? – *Wondering Woman*

Hi Wondering Woman!

Yes! Consider the following example: Patty was at a work event talking to her colleagues when her husband sauntered up next to her to join the conversation. He casually rested his hand on her lower back in a way that seemed ordinary. However, unbeknownst to him, she became turned on by the way he was gently stroking her back. She found his touches unexpectedly erotic, but he was oblivious to that fact. Thus, it was romantic to her but not to him.

Of course, he was quite pleased when, after a few minutes, she leaned further into him, arching her back in pleasure . . . before excusing the both of them from the conversation. Their walk to the car was slowed by her stopping to kiss him—passionately—several times!

***

Dear Beth: I'm a sapiosexual, someone who's turned on by intelligence. I just can't be with a partner who doesn't keep up with me intellectually, so I think "intellectual intimacy" is imperative. Why don't you talk about that? —*Interested in Intellect*

Hi Interested in Intellect!

Great question! Thanks for bringing this up. A lot of people have asked me about this, so I'm grateful for a reminder to address it.

I also consider myself a sapiosexual, yet I've realized that being attracted to and/or turned on by something like intelligence doesn't necessarily require intimacy. For example, I know a lot of people who are attracted to athletes, but that doesn't mean they need athletic intimacy. While I am being somewhat flippant here, I do understand your point.

Allow me to tell you about my client Shellie. She's a brilliant chemist with a list of publications a mile long. She worried that she would never meet anyone as smart as she is, which was not an unreasonable fear. Fortunately, when she met Mel, with his above-average but less-than-genius level of intelligence, and he became the great love of her life, she discovered that their difference in IQ scores didn't matter at all. Shellie realized that what she actually needed was someone who understood and respected her passionate dedication to chemistry. When Shellie came home from work at night, she didn't need to discuss the specifics of her work; she'd spent all day talking about those things with colleagues. The look on her face when I asked how intimately connected she felt to those colleagues was priceless, by the way.

In short, Shellie wanted a partner who was intellectually curious. What she *needed* was someone willing to be emotionally intimate with her so they would empathize with her frustrations with the bureaucracy surrounding her funding, her difficulty recruiting the best fellows, even her exuberance that a paper she'd been slaving over for months was finally accepted for publication.

In other words, *intellectual connection* is great and may be a requirement for your partner choice, but generally, it isn't a required building block for successful relationships.

***

Dear Beth: My husband lost his job several months ago, so I've been working as much overtime as I can to keep things going for our family. It's been incredibly stressful for both of us, but I try not to complain because I don't want to make it worse for him.

The problem is, with everything going on, we barely see each other, never go out, and only talk about family stuff. I still love him; I just don't have the energy for sex these days. But my husband wants sex more now than he did when he was working. He's upset that I keep saying no, which pisses me off because I'm killing myself trying to keep us afloat financially. It's not his fault that he lost his job, but I think it's unreasonable for him to be demanding sex right now.

I know you think sex is important to a relationship, but don't you think I deserve a break? – *Feeling Exhausted*

Hi Feeling Exhausted!

You certainly deserve a break! And a round of applause for stepping up for your family. Truly. I can tell you are giving your all, and it's not easy. Much respect to you, my friend. I hope your husband finds a new job sooner rather than later so your burden is lessened quickly.

That being said, I think your husband is also suffering. While he's asking for sex, I suspect there's actually much more to it.

I've worked with thousands of men, and what almost all of them have in common is that they rely on their jobs to "prove" their value. In other words, when things are going well at work, they feel successful.

166

When they lose their job, they feel like a loser. More specifically, they feel as if they're "less of a man." (By this I mean they tend to judge themselves, or fear judgment from others, based on society's still prevalent stereotype/expectation for males.)

Sadly, it's also common for a man to feel further emasculated by having to financially rely on his wife. After all, most of us are taught that a "good man" is one who is gainfully employed, provides for his family, and is financially responsible. (A "good woman" is generally thought to be one who's attractive, attentive to her appearance, family-oriented, and supportive of others.)

To be fair, it's usually not because a man doesn't admire, respect, and appreciate his wife for stepping up. It's just that he feels guilty that she has to do so. Subconsciously, he may also be fearful that she'll realize she doesn't "need" him, which is tantamount to his feeling impotent.

While on the surface, men tend to pretend they're handling things calmly, deep down they can be flailing like a drowning person. When they're desperate to prove their worth, their "manliness," it's typical for men to seek validation through the only other socially approved means available to them: sex.

When sexually engaged, men are finally able to let their guard down. For a man, being desired by—and being able to sexually satisfy—his partner can be the reminder he needs to believe that he is a "good man," even if he doesn't have a job. (As a divorce lawyer, I saw too many marriages end because, in the midst of professional upheaval, the husband sought affirmation from someone other than his spouse.)

So now, here you both are: He's feeling "less than." You're doing "more than." He's a man trying to get his needs for affirmation met through sex. You're a woman who feels that's unreasonable because since you are not getting your emotional needs met, you don't have the energy to meet his needs.

While it's a painful circle, akin to the question of whether the chicken or the egg comes first, it's an absolutely common one. I hope that reading this book and doing the exercises will help you find mutually satisfying ways to give each other what you want.

***

Dear Beth: You mentioned there would be a State of Your Union assessment later in this book. That makes me nervous! What if I fail it? Or what if my relationship does? – *Nervous Nelly*

Hi Nervous Nelly!

I've got some terrific news: There is no way to fail the assessment! The only "failure" I see is doing nothing while a good relationship goes bad.

This assessment isn't about judgment. It's a gift of clarity—the ability to see what is, where your strengths are, where you want to improve, and where you overlap or differ in perspectives. Most important of all, it will give you a "marker" by which to measure your growth so you can celebrate how far you've come instead of being overwhelmed by the endless journey ahead.

Remember, we want your relationship to be a journey interesting enough to last a lifetime—not a quick trip to the nearest vista where you'll stay for years, becoming so bored, you'll be excited for death!

As long as you answer honestly, you're gonna be golden. Even though you'll be asked to write down several numbers, keep in mind there's no score that is "bad" or "wrong." It's all just information to help you create the relationship you truly desire.

You should also take comfort in the fact that once you take the assessment, you can move on to a section of tangible, practical, actionable exercises that will help improve things. These practices aren't Band-Aids. They're not superficial fixes. They get to the heart of things, which means they've got the power to transform your relationship.

So without further ado, let's get crackin'. No stress—it's time to assess!

Tantalizing Takeaways

- There is no way to "fail" the State of Your Union assessment—as long as you're reading this book and putting what you've learned into practice, you're succeeding!
- Remember that there will be times in your relationship when one intimacy (or two, or three!) is present or stronger than the others. And just like you can drive for a short time with a flat tire, the key is to repair it before the other tires are permanently damaged.
- An annual relationship review is the best way to ensure that your happy, healthy relationship lasts.

Check Check . . . the State of Your Union

Woo-hoo! You made it! Now's the time you've been waiting for, the moment when we get really personal, as we zero in on . . .

You.

Your partner.

And your relationship.

As we start assessing where intimacy flourishes (or doesn't) in *your* relationship, this would be a great time to get your partner involved if you haven't already.

You might be sweating bullets right now. Maybe, as the spotlight hits you, you find yourself thinking, *Yikes, I'm not ready for this level of scrutiny!* Maybe you're tempted to casually slide this book onto your bedside table, where it will soon enter the coaster stage, attracting a nice layer of dust.

Before you do so, though, let me ask you a question:

Why do people prioritize and invest in car maintenance but not relationship maintenance?

> Why do people prioritize and invest in car maintenance but not relationship maintenance?

People are able to understand that failure to change the oil in a vehicle isn't good for the engine, even though the car still runs. The most coveted cars require *lots* of care, attention, and money to keep them in good shape, but their owners proudly defend them, arguing that they're completely worth it. In fact, if someone lets a Ferrari fall into disrepair—or even just get dirty!—they will be shamed for showing a lack of regard for something so valuable.

Isn't your relationship truly one of the most valuable parts of your life?

Isn't it reasonable to care for your relationship *at least* as well as your car?

If you want your relationship to thrive, you need to constantly concoct new ideas, seek expert insights, and conduct regular checkups. The following State of Your Union assessment is the only tool you'll need for a lifetime of checkups. It will help you gather the information and insight you need to nurture your relationship.

See? That's not so scary, right?

So here you go . . .

State of Your Union Assessment

You may use this to evaluate your relationship with yourself and/or a partner. However, my suggestion is to perform a self-assessment before you perform a relationship assessment.

If you're employing this assessment alone, substitute "self" for "partner" and ignore the question about how you think the other person feels.

If you're partnered, each of you should answer these questions in writing privately before any joint discussion. Once you've both completed the assessment, it's helpful to share your responses with each other.

Whether you use this alone or with a partner, the key is to accept all answers without judgment or antagonism. This is about gaining insight into how one perceives things; there is no right or wrong. You'll gain more if you focus on understanding the feelings behind the answers rather than trying to convince anyone (including yourself) to feel differently. Clarity and insight are the goals because they're what you need to be able to improve things.

I've included two blank copies of the State of Your Union worksheet but be sure to make a few more copies of the pages. This way, you can revisit it every few months and take stock of how the perspective about your relationship has changed as you and your partner have continued to do the work in this book.

State Of OUR UNION

NAMES:_____ DATE: _____

Rank each of these on a scale from 1-10 (10 being *amazing*) as they relate to your relationship from your perspective.

		1	2	3	4	5	6	7	8	9	10
01	Physical Intimacy	○	○	○	○	○	○	○	○	○	○
02	Emotional Intimacy	○	○	○	○	○	○	○	○	○	○
03	Sexual Intimacy	○	○	○	○	○	○	○	○	○	○
04	Romantic Intimacy	○	○	○	○	○	○	○	○	○	○
05	Spiritual Intimacy	○	○	○	○	○	○	○	○	○	○
06	Overall love for _____	○	○	○	○	○	○	○	○	○	○
07	How in love I am with _____	○	○	○	○	○	○	○	○	○	○
08	Overall level of "happiness" I feel with our relationship	○	○	○	○	○	○	○	○	○	○
09	Overall level of "happiness" I think my partner feels	○	○	○	○	○	○	○	○	○	○
10	How committed am I to investing in our relationship right now	○	○	○	○	○	○	○	○	○	○

State Of
OUR UNION

NOTES

RESOLVED:

State Of OUR UNION

NAMES:_____ DATE: _____

**Rank each of these on a scale from 1-10 (10 being *amazing*)
as they relate to your relationship from your perspective.**

		1	2	3	4	5	6	7	8	9	10
01	Physical Intimacy	○	○	○	○	○	○	○	○	○	○
02	Emotional Intimacy	○	○	○	○	○	○	○	○	○	○
03	Sexual Intimacy	○	○	○	○	○	○	○	○	○	○
04	Romantic Intimacy	○	○	○	○	○	○	○	○	○	○
05	Spiritual Intimacy	○	○	○	○	○	○	○	○	○	○
06	Overall love for _____	○	○	○	○	○	○	○	○	○	○
07	How in love I am with _____	○	○	○	○	○	○	○	○	○	○
08	Overall level of "happiness" I feel with our relationship	○	○	○	○	○	○	○	○	○	○
09	Overall level of "happiness" I think my partner feels	○	○	○	○	○	○	○	○	○	○
10	How committed am I to investing in our relationship right now	○	○	○	○	○	○	○	○	○	○

State Of
OUR UNION

NOTES

RESOLVED:

Bravo! You did it!

Here's what I see in you:

1. You are brave enough to declare, in no uncertain terms, that your relationship is important to you.
2. You are confident enough to examine yourself and your relationship carefully, knowing you can handle whatever you uncover.
3. You possess great power, which you are willing to use to make changes in order to make life healthier, happier, and more joyous.
4. You are destined for great and lasting love.

No matter what you've learned from the assessment, whether things are fabulous or need lots of improvement, it's time for you to have some fun! You deserve to cut loose while creating intimacy galore using the Practical Playbook in Part Two.

Get ready. Get set. Now go get intimate!

Tantalizing Takeaways

- Love doesn't require perfection, nor is it perfect. It does require courage though.
- Take the State of Your Union assessment at least once a year to check in with yourself and/or your relationship with your partner.
- If you're afraid to share your honest responses with your partner, commit to the Intimacy Practices for a month or two before doing so.

PART TWO

A Practical Playbook: Easy Intimacy Practices for Everyone

Welcome to the fun part. You made it!

On the pages that follow, you'll find a number of practices to explore alone and/or with your partner.

Each of these practices will create at least one kind of intimacy; many will create two or more. With practice, I expect you'll find each of the practices capable of inspiring all 5 intimacies.

Some may stir up intimacies you'd never expect them to.

Some may stir up other things, in which case you'll get to enjoy some "side effects" (wink wink).

There's no wrong way to embark on these practices—as long as you approach them with an open mind and heart. My recommended approach would be to start with the first one and work your way through each one in order from there. I have purposefully placed what might be considered the "easier" exercises upfront. This serves a purpose: getting you and your partner comfortable together.

The big win is for you to play, recognize, and, hopefully, surprise yourself.

And guess what?

You can enjoy multiple intimacies!

No recovery period required. ;)

After each practice, I have included a worksheet so that you can record your thoughts after that practice is performed. Each sheet offers space for up to five entries, so that over time you can notice how you and your partner's feelings change over time. This will truly allow you to both become more in tune with what you each like.

Intimacy Practice 1

How We Do Intimacy

List five of your favorite ways, with specific examples, to experience
each kind of intimacy. (Examples: **Physical intimacy:** I like a
two-minute hug in the morning before my coffee. **Sexual intimacy:** I
get aroused when you kiss my neck when I'm sitting at the dinner table.)

Ask your partner to do the same. Share your answers with each
other so you know how best to connect. Then commit to doing at least
one thing daily from your partner's worksheets.

I've included two copies per person of this worksheet but make more
if needed.

YOUR NAME: _____

Physical Intimacy
1. _____
2. _____
3. _____
4. _____
5. _____

Emotional Intimacy
1. _____
2. _____
3. _____
4. _____
5. _____

Sexual Intimacy
1. _____
2. _____
3. _____
4. _____
5. _____

Romantic Intimacy
1. _____
2. _____
3. _____
4. _____
5. _____

Spiritual Intimacy
1. _____
2. _____
3. _____
4. _____
5. _____

PARTNER NAME: _____

Physical Intimacy

    1. _____
    2. _____
    3. _____
    4. _____
    5. _____

Emotional Intimacy

    1. _____
    2. _____
    3. _____
    4. _____
    5. _____

Sexual Intimacy

    1. _____
    2. _____
    3. _____
    4. _____
    5. _____

Romantic Intimacy

    1. _____
    2. _____
    3. _____
    4. _____
    5. _____

Spiritual Intimacy

    1. _____
    2. _____
    3. _____
    4. _____
    5. _____

YOUR NAME: _____

Physical Intimacy

1. _____
2. _____
3. _____
4. _____
5. _____

Emotional Intimacy

1. _____
2. _____
3. _____
4. _____
5. _____

Sexual Intimacy

1. _____
2. _____
3. _____
4. _____
5. _____

Romantic Intimacy

1. _____
2. _____
3. _____
4. _____
5. _____

Spiritual Intimacy

1. _____
2. _____
3. _____
4. _____
5. _____

PARTNER NAME: _____

Physical Intimacy
1. _____
2. _____
3. _____
4. _____
5. _____

Emotional Intimacy
1. _____
2. _____
3. _____
4. _____
5. _____

Sexual Intimacy
1. _____
2. _____
3. _____
4. _____
5. _____

Romantic Intimacy
1. _____
2. _____
3. _____
4. _____
5. _____

Spiritual Intimacy
1. _____
2. _____
3. _____
4. _____
5. _____

Intimacy Practice 2

Face Cupping

THE QUICKIE BOX

HOW: Use your hands to gently, intentionally, cup your lover's face.

WHY: Simple acts of physical touch create comfort, warmth, and love.

In recent years, cupping therapy has become even more popular in the United States. This is a form of alternative medicine in which heated cups are applied to the skin to create a suction effect.

That is *not* the kind of cupping I'm talking about. For this kind of cup, you only need your own two hands. In fact, before you try cupping your partner's face, I'd like you to try this exercise on yourself.

Take a moment to get comfortable. Sit somewhere cozy. Shake out any leftover jitters. Inhale deeply.

Now put your hands under your own chin in a V shape—cup your face gently.

Don't rush it. It might feel silly at first but see if you can relax into it. Let your fingers rest comfortably against your cheeks.

Now imagine love flowing from your heart through your chest to your left arm, up to your hand, to your fingers. Feel it flow seamlessly into your face, where its warmth relaxes you. Notice your own tenderness, your ease or discomfort, as well as any other feelings, whether they're physical or emotional. Breathe deeply and slowly as the love exits your face through the fingers on your right hand, returning to your heart, where the cycle begins again. Allow yourself to not only notice but also to savor the comfort, warmth, and love of your own touch.

All too often, we forget that we have the power to soothe ourselves. Let this be your reminder.

The power of this simple exercise can surprise people, especially those with a tough exterior. The effects are magnified by looking at yourself in the mirror while doing the exercise. It's not unusual for clients to burst into tears.

Next time you're having a rough day or totally losing your sh*t, step out of the fray, just for a minute, to cup your face. It's one of the most effective and efficient ways to ground yourself, or someone else, that I've ever experienced.

I've even used this technique with children when they're having a hard time. I look them in the eye while gently cupping their face and assuring them that I'm here for them. It creates a calm zone of safety within which we can regroup.

When doing this exercise with your partner or anyone else, ask them if they'll allow you a minute to love them (and wink if you need to!). Then look them in the eyes and ask if it's okay for you to touch their face. (This slow, deliberate start is actually powerful. Requiring their agreement brings their focus to the moment, making it difficult for them to ignore your touch or disassociate by thinking about other stuff.)

> Silence keeps the focus on the physical sensations that connect you.

Take a moment, if necessary, to warm or cool your hands before placing them gently under your partner's chin with your fingers against their cheeks. You might feel an urge to talk, but I encourage you not to do so. Silence keeps the focus on the physical sensations that connect you. Allow each breath to circulate your love through your body and into theirs. Before removing your hands, give notice by suggesting you both take one last deep breath and notice all the love flowing between you. Feel free to hug or kiss afterward as a "closing."

I love how easy and intimate face cupping is. I also relish the fact that it's not inherently sexual, but it *can* be. Incorporating this kind of intense, loving touch into your relationship makes a big impact. (If you doubt the bonding effect, I dare you to try it with someone you don't care for. I'm guessing that idea is as appalling to you as it is to me—which I think proves my point.)

If you're not used to pleasurable physical intimacy or the emotional intimacy that comes from looking someone in the eyes, it can take a big effort to get comfortable with this. If this exercise makes you really uncomfortable, here's a tip: Close your eyes. But don't give up, because you probably have a lot to gain from practicing it regularly.

Suggested frequency? Every day!

Bonus? Once you start touching, it's likely that the rest of your body will start itching to be touched as well! After all, your body, your skin, craves pleasurable sensations.

Don't deprive yourself any longer.

Remember: at the end of each practice, I've added a page where you can record your notes after each time performing the practice, up to five total times. (If you want more, make a copy and add the loose sheet to the book!)

First Time:

_____

_____

_____

Second Time:

_____

_____

_____

Third Time:

_____

_____

_____

Fourth Time:

_____

_____

_____

Fifth Time:

_____

_____

_____

Intimacy Practice 3

Standing Spoons

THE QUICKIE BOX

HOW: Two partners spoon standing up, one person's back against the other's chest.

WHY: As you lean into each other for support, it gives you both comfort as well as a shared perspective.

Who doesn't love a big bear hug, right? Wrong!

Sure, lots of people do, but others aren't as enthusiastic. In a recent study, psychologists found that people raised by parents who were frequent huggers were much more likely to be huggers in adulthood, compared with the children of non-hugging parents, who expressed greater discomfort when hugged.[44]

Maybe you and your partner both love hugs. Fantastic! I give you my full blessing to up the hug quotient in your relationship.

But this exercise is good for huggers and non-huggers alike.

---

[44] Melissa Locker, "Why Some People Hate Being Hugged, According to Science," *Time*, September 4, 2018, https://time.com/5379586/people-hate-hugged-science/.

I'm sure you've got the idea already since the name of this exercise says it all. But all that's required is to spoon while standing with one person's back against the other's chest. The arms of the one in back are wrapped around the front of the other. The front spoon uses their arms to cover the other's.

This position not only gives both of you a sense of comfort in that you can lean on or into each other for support, but it also gives you a shared sense of perspective, a sense of solidarity. You stand together, supporting one another, while seeing things from the same position. This creates a subconscious belief that your perspective is aligned, which fosters a deep sense of connection.

This is a fantastic way to appreciate a sunset or a view from a balcony or to face a stressful situation.

Standing Spoons is a way of hugging that allows you to feel intimately connected to your partner while still being able to focus on the world around you.

First Time:

_____

_____

_____

Second Time:

_____

_____

_____

Third Time:

_____

_____

_____

Fourth Time:

_____

_____

_____

Fifth Time:

_____

_____

_____

Intimacy Practice 4

Kick-Ass Compliments

THE QUICKIE BOX

HOW: Craft every compliment with unique, specific details,
using more words to express your feelings fully.

WHY: Sincere compliments are a free, endlessly renewable power source
that can create emotional, sexual, romantic, and even spiritual intimacy.

D id you get that?
Let me say it again, just in case:

**Sincere compliments are a free, endlessly renewable
power source that can create emotional, sexual,
romantic, and even spiritual intimacy.**

How many times have you given compliments, only to have them brushed aside as if they mean nothing?

Do you or your partner say things along the lines of "It's not even worth saying nice things because they either don't pay attention or don't believe me"?

If this is you, I feel ya. But I hate it because compliments are too valuable to be wasted.

I truly believe that sincere compliments are precious gifts that should be shared generously; each one deserves a warm reception along with a kind acknowledgment. To a giver of compliments, it can feel almost insulting if the recipient doesn't value your offering, even if your brain tells you it's about their own insecurities, not about you.

I want to help you give your compliments the best chance of "success," meaning the recipient can't help but pay attention to it.

Here's all you need to know:

**The secret sauce for kick-ass compliments
is as simple as *being specific*.**

Yep, that's pretty much it. (Well, of course, be sincere and authentic, not slimy or patronizing—but that should be a given!)

Why is specificity so important?

Because including details, reasoning, and your *why* gives more of a complete story, which is hard to brush off. It also stops others from imagining their own version of your story.

Here's an example:

> Wife says, "Thanks for buying the new lawn mower. I'm sure it'll make it easier for you."
>
> Husband hears her words, but to his mind, they aren't the whole story, so he fills in the gaps, which include an underlying accusation: "Why haven't you used it yet?" The sad part is he doesn't even recognize that the story is of his own making, so in annoyance, he brushes off the nice words with a "Yeah, right."
>
> Wife is then not only miffed but also thoroughly confused because what she meant was, "I hate dealing

with the yard, and I'm so glad I can count on you to take care of it."

Do you see how a compliment can go wrong?

We can learn a lot from the character of Brad in *The Rocky Horror Picture Show,* who gave Janet a compliment about her bouquet-catching skills that stuck because it was too specific to brush off.

The only thing I would suggest he add would be an explanation of *why* he's giving her this compliment by saying something like, "I admire that you are willing to take what you want."

This is important because we want to know whether compliments come with strings or not. It's like gifts: We need to understand the terms before we accept them. Women, in particular, are very sensitive to men's using compliments as an attempt to initiate sexual intimacy. Whether this is the man's intention or a story made up by the recipient of the compliment is hard to determine . . . unless the compliment is specific and explicit. (I don't mean raunchy—rather, in a way that clarifies the giver's intention behind the compliment.) For example, I love giving strangers compliments, but I want to alleviate any concern about my intentions, so I might say, "Sorry for staring at you as you were walking, but I think your shoes are fabulous! They're the perfect color for your outfit, and I think you deserve to know that you're rockin' it today."

The next time you want to give a compliment that sticks so that it will be received as the gift you intend it to be, use more words to provide a complete story so nothing gets lost or added in translation.

Instead of saying, "I love you," try saying, "I love you because talking to you makes me feel like I can be successful, even when things are tough. I needed this pep talk today; I'm touched that you made time for me when I needed you. I know you're busy now though, so I'll let you get back to work."

If you want to spark some sexy flames, you might be inclined to say, "I can't wait to have sex with you tonight." However, you'll probably get a more exciting response if you expand a bit, like, "Damn, I know you're busy tonight, but I can't seem to get any work done because all I'm thinking about is your legs in those heels you're wearing today. I just don't know how I'm going to be able to keep my hands to myself tonight."

Here are a couple of other examples:

"You have great boobs."

vs.

"Your amazing boobs just popped into my mind, and now I can't stop thinking about them! They're so much fun to touch with my hands, my face, my mouth . . ."

"You're great."

vs.

"I want you. I want to be so close to you. I literally want to be inside you and feel your warmth." (Hello again, King Charles and Camilla!)

"You're so strong."

vs.

"I so appreciate that you're willing and strong enough to do the heavy lifting for me. It makes me feel taken care of and makes me want to take care of you."

By the way, don't think that it's just women who ignore compliments, and don't think that anyone is so confident that they don't "need" to hear more nice things about themselves!

Remember, compliments, when well crafted, are a free, endlessly renewable power source, capable of uplifting both giver and receiver while also creating intimacy.

First Time:

_____

_____

_____

Second Time:

_____

_____

_____

Third Time:

_____

_____

_____

Fourth Time:

_____

_____

_____

Fifth Time:

_____

_____

_____

Intimacy Practice 5

How to Talk 101
(a.k.a. The Art of a Meaningful Conversation)

THE QUICKIE BOX

HOW: Use the **4 Es** (embrace, engage, empathize, encourage) to ensure fulfilling conversations before you ask if your help is wanted.

WHY: Men and women generally have very different communication styles. Frequently, this can leave people dissatisfied after important conversations, despite good intentions.

Some of us have spent our whole lives relying on personal, emotional conversations to forge relationships. Others have spent their whole lives avoiding them.

One of the most helpful discoveries I made after working with thousands of couples is that men and women have grown up with very different rules of etiquette when it comes to conversations.

From the time they are boys, males are taught to speak up frequently, loudly, for as long as they want. In a group of men, it's assumed that anyone who has something to say will say it. Men assume that if someone is quiet, it's because they don't have anything to say.

Girls, on the other hand, are taught to politely speak only after being acknowledged by the authority figure or person in charge. (You probably remember boys blurting out answers in elementary school, but can you remember any girls doing so?) Girls are discouraged from raising their voices to speak over someone, mocked if they're "too" confident, and ridiculed or hushed for speaking too long. This continues into adulthood when, even in professional settings, women are expected to offer opinions rather than state facts or conclusions and, most importantly, to seek agreement from the group or authority figure.

In general, women learn to limit the frequency of their contributions to a conversation while also deliberately passing the (figurative) mic before anyone accuses them of hogging the spotlight. (This is especially true when men are present, which may help you understand why women often prefer to sit together even when out with other couples.) It's common for women in a group setting to remain quiet until they are invited to speak. Even then, a woman is likely to apologize for giving a complete answer, ending with "Enough about me; I'm sorry to have gone on so long! Please tell me what you think about . . ."

If you know me, you're probably rolling your eyes because I have a reputation for being outspoken (wink!). I won't pretend to argue that reality, but I will tell you that I am incredibly sensitive to the fact I may be the only woman actively participating in a conversation in a coed group. I hate that I feel pressure to "pass the mic" rather than being comfortable in taking my time to say what I want to say and that I hesitate to speak up too often lest I be deemed aggressive. Years ago, someone with whom I'd attended law school said, "Oh, I remember you! You were the one in class who was always debating the professors." I don't think that was intended as a compliment. All this to say, men and women carry different baggage, even if you don't notice it.

Back to the matter at hand: improving conversations for mutual benefit.

Obviously, it's problematic that men and women are operating under two very different sets of expectations during conversations, which often results in women feeling unheard while their partner is thinking, *Well, you should have spoken up!*

I'm not suggesting either of these paradigms is right or wrong. Either approach is workable. What I am saying is that meaningful conversations between people operating under different paradigms are not likely to be rewarding.

After witnessing the frustration felt by so many men—hearing them confess that they have no idea how to talk to women (even if they love them dearly)—I started breaking things down in a way that makes it easier to have more satisfying conversations. I make no apologies for the fact that this approach is specifically designed to accommodate those who hesitate to speak up. However, I assure you that it's applicable to conversations between anyone because it ensures empathy, which all of us crave.

The following steps provide a straightforward structure for meaningful, intimate conversations with anyone you want to connect with.

Here's how to have a meaningful conversation with your partner in five easy steps:

1. **Embrace** their desire for conversation. Do this by carving out time to spend with them when you won't be rushed, in a setting that allows you to focus on them without constant interruptions. For some additional ideas, see The Love Seat: Home of the Cuddle Huddle exercise (Intimacy Practice 13). Note: If talking isn't generally your thing, take pleasure in the fact that they want to connect with you.

2. **Engage** by asking questions to not only start the conversation but to also delve deeper throughout.

3. **Empathize** by affirming what the other person is saying. "That really *does* suck! I would have been pissed. I don't know how you stayed so calm!" etc. Caution: *Don't lie!* Having empathy doesn't mean you would feel or act the same way, only that you understand their perspective, for example, "I know how much you loved those shoes (or golf clubs, etc.); of course you're furious that they were stolen!"

4. **Encourage** them to talk as long as they want or need to, even if they offer to self-police their time, e.g., "No, go on. This is important to you, so it's important to me. I'm not in a hurry. What happened next?" Questions such as "How did you keep your cool?" and "Did you want to hit someone?" and "How did they respond?" and "How do you feel now?" will encourage your partner to continue sharing. Don't worry thinking that your encouragement will make things drag on; it will simply allow the conversation to feel complete to your partner. It may seem like forever to you, but that's probably an indication that you previously cut off conversations before your partner was finished. When they're done, when they feel sated, their response to your encouragement will likely be along the lines of, "Thanks, I needed that, but I'm ready to move on now." The most amazing thing is they probably will be able to do so now since they not only unburdened themselves but they also got to bask in your undivided attention. It's a double whammy!

After employing the 4 Es, take a well-deserved pause! This might be a great time for a hug, sympathetic pat, or other physical expression of support.

But *wait!* You haven't fixed anything, right? Yay!! I know it's hard to suppress the need to fix things, but now that your partner has talked it all out, you've got a better chance of them accepting or at least appreciating your offer of assistance.

5. **Ask** your partner how they want you to support them. Did they just need to vent? Do they need you to be upset and angry too? Do they want to cry while you hold them? Are they looking for a reality check? Or do they want you to problem-solve with them or fix it on your own? This is important: Don't offer solutions or instructions unless or until they want them. Feel free to say, "I know you're perfectly capable and that you don't *need* me to fix your problems, but I like contributing to your happiness by helping you in whatever way I can." (Beware of the fact that this might make them melt into tears . . . or your arms.)

Lastly, offer them the option to revisit this issue at any time. Also, remind them that your offer to help remains open.

First Time:

_____
_____
_____

Second Time:

_____
_____
_____

Third Time:

_____
_____
_____

Fourth Time:

_____
_____
_____

Fifth Time:

_____
_____
_____

Intimacy Practice 6

Just Say NO!

For those who struggle with boundaries, hate saying *no* because they don't want to disappoint anyone, or hate hearing *no* because the rejection is too painful, here's a fun exercise:

Every day, ask your partner or anyone else five random questions to which the answer will absolutely be *no* but that won't upset or affect either of you.

Here are some to try:

- Would you like to adopt a pet tiger?
- Would you like to sleep on the roof together?
- Will you move to a deserted island with me?

- Can we spend all our savings on the lottery this weekend?
- Will you have sex with me in the stadium, on the bleachers, where everyone can see us, during the football game?

Enjoy laughing together at the outrageousness of the questions you come up with.

When you receive the *no,* thank your partner for the respect they showed you in giving you an honest answer. At the same time, applaud yourself for being strong enough to weather another *no.*

And maybe don't tell them you've got the tiger waiting in the car.

First Time:

_____

_____

_____

Second Time:

_____

_____

_____

Third Time:

_____

_____

_____

Fourth Time:

_____

_____

_____

Fifth Time:

_____

_____

_____

Intimacy Practice 7

How to Become
Fluent in Feelings
(No Language Class Required!)

THE QUICKIE BOX

HOW: Use the list of emotions to help you identify
and explain what you're feeling.

WHY: Expressing your feelings more specifically
makes emotional intimacy easier, which increases
the likelihood that you'll get what you need.

Not all words have some deep, magical meaning. Words can be empty. Conversations can be pointless. There are countless couples who talk to each other plenty, yet still have zero idea how the other person actually feels.

If you're into efficiency, using words to express your feelings can be a shortcut to emotional intimacy.

Sounds simple, like something we should have learned when we were kids, right? But instead, what you probably learned was to ignore or override your feelings because they are annoying, if not to you, then to those around you.

You're probably a good learner, which means, unfortunately, you excelled at this lesson. And today, you might have problems talking about any feelings, not just the "problematic" ones. Men, you might even have had this lesson beaten into you.

Please know that I'm with ya, but I promise you that life is actually easier when you're in touch with your feelings. Otherwise, they become like invisible gremlins, fighting for control of your life.

As a recovering non-feeler, I know you can learn to make things better for yourself, so stick with me, please.

If you're not sure what a non-feeler is, it's someone who responds to a loved one who extends a sincere "How are you?" like this: "I'm fine. Just recovering from a crash with an eighteen-wheeler, but no biggie. How are you?"

Well, um . . . Okay, then . . .

I hate receiving responses like this because I have no idea how to respond. I'm thinking that crashing into an eighteen-wheeler is a terribly scary event, but they're acting like it's nothing. Does that mean I'm being melodramatic if I express concern for their well-being? Am I being invasive if I ask if they're hurt? Does this mean they don't want to talk about it? Am I supposed to ignore what would appear to be a major event?

Yeah. It's hard talking to non-feelers. At least with feelers, you know what's going on without having to second-guess yourself.

Healthy, happy people learn to face their emotions in real time. *You* can learn to do this too.

Much like developing physical intimacy, learning to recognize and name your emotions can be strange or uncomfortable if it's not something you normally do. Thankfully, much like physical intimacy, it also gets easier with practice.

I've included an extensive (but not exhaustive) list of emotions below. Whenever you sense a feeling, you can refer to this list to find the right emotions to describe it.

List of Emotions

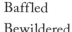

Acceptance
Admiration
Adoration
Affection
Afraid
Agitation
Agony
Aggressive
Alarm
Alarmed
Alienation
Amazement
Ambivalence
Amusement
Anger
Anguish
Annoyed
Anticipating
Anxious
Apathy
Apoplectic
Appreciative
Apprehension
Arrogant
Assertive
Astonished
Attentiveness
Attraction
Aversion

Baffled
Bewildered
Bitter
Bittersweetness
Bliss
Bored
Brazen
Brooding
Calm
Carefree
Careless
Caring
Charity
Cheeky
Cheerfulness
Claustrophobic
Coercive
Comfortable
Confident
Confusion
Contempt
Content
Courage
Cowardly
Cruelty
Curiosity
Cynicism
Dazed
Dejection

Delighted
Demoralized
Depressed
Desire
Despair
Determined
Disappointment
Disbelief
Discombobulated
Discomfort
Discontentment
Disgruntled
Disgust
Disheartened
Dislike
Dismay
Disoriented
Dispirited
Displeasure
Distraction
Distress
Disturbed
Dominant
Doubt
Dread
Driven
Dumbstruck
Eagerness
Ecstasy

Elation

Embarrassment

Empathy

Enchanted

Enlightened

Ennui

Enraged

Enthusiasm

Envy

Epiphany

Euphoria

Exasperated

Excitement

Expectancy

Fascination

Fear

Flakey

Focused

Fondness

Friendliness

Fright

Frustrated

Fuming

Fury

Glee

Gloomy

Glumness

Gratitude

Greed

Grief

Grouchy

Grumpy

Guilt

Happy

Hatred

Helpless

Homesick

Hopeful

Hopeless

Horrified

Hospitable

Humiliated

Humble

Hurt

Hysteria

Hyper

Idleness

Impatient

Indifference

Indignant

Infatuation

Infuriated

Insecurity

Insightful

Insulted

Interest

Intrigued

Irritated

Isolated

Jealousy

Joviality

Joy

Jubilation

Kind

Lazy

Liking

Livid

Loathing

Lonely

Longing

Loopy

Love

Lust

Mad

Melancholy

Miserable

Miserliness

Mixed up

Modesty

Moody

Mortified

Mystified

Nasty

Nauseated

Negative

Neglect

Nervous

Nostalgic

Numb

Obstinate

Offended

Optimistic

Outrage

Overwhelmed

Panicked

Paranoid

Passion

Patience

Pensiveness

Perplexed
Persevering
Pessimism
Pissed
Pity
Pleased
Pleasure
Politeness
Positive
Possessive
Powerless
Pride
Puzzled
Rage
Rash
Rattled
Regret
Rejected
Relaxed
Relieved
Reluctant
Remorse
Resentment
Resignation
Restlessness
Revulsion
Ruthless
Sadness
Satisfaction
Scared
Scorn
Seething
Self-caring

Self-compassionate
Self-confident
Self-conscious
Self-critical
Self-loathing
Self-motivated
Self-pity
Self-respecting
Self-understanding
Sentimentality
Serenity
Shame
Shameless
Shocked
Smug
Sorrow
Spite
Stressed
Strong
Stubborn
Stuck
Submissive
Suffering
Sullenness
Surprise
Suspense
Suspicious
Sympathy
Tenderness
Tension
Terror
Thankfulness
Thrilled

Tired
Tolerance
Torment
Triumphant
Troubled
Trust
Uncertainty
Undermined
Uneasiness
Unhappy
Unnerved
Unsettled
Unsure
Upset
Vengeful
Vicious
Vigilant
Vulnerable
Weak
Woe
Worried
Worthy
Wrath

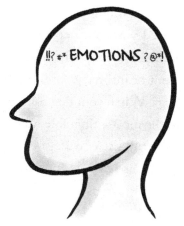

217

This exercise may seem silly, but it has helped a lot of people, including me. Feel free to laugh with yourself and all of us who had to learn the language of feelings, just like we had to learn algebra—*painfully!* (Look, that's a feeling! Yay, me!)

Heads up: Getting your kids or friends to join you in this exercise makes it a lot of fun. It can even be a drinking game if you want. (Maybe only if you've got adult kids though!)

One way or another, *practice.*

When something happens to you, when a feeling wells up inside you, pay attention. Express it out loud to yourself: "When I turned in my big project at work, I felt really proud. I felt gratified. I felt relieved. I'd spent a lot of time on it, which the client acknowledged. That made me feel great, successful, as though I had impressed them."

There are layers and layers of emotion beneath every one of our experiences; life gets richer as you begin to notice them.

As you become more fluent in feelings, you'll find it easier to connect in a meaningful way with those around you, which will make it easier for you to create more emotional intimacy, *especially* with the person you love.

"When I woke up this morning," you might say, "I looked at you asleep beside me, with your hair spilling over the pillow. I felt so good and safe with you. I'm happy to be sharing this life with you."

You might be scared it will sound weird or awkward or corny, scared your partner will ridicule you for telling them what you felt. Vulnerability is inherently risky, which is exactly why it's a key ingredient of intimacy. Amusingly enough, this is where we can learn from dogs. When your dog rolls onto her back, belly up, she's exposing herself in the most vulnerable way she knows, but that's what it takes to get the belly rub she craves.

Be as brave as your dog; be vulnerable with those you love.

First Time:

_____

_____

_____

Second Time:

_____

_____

_____

Third Time:

_____

_____

_____

Fourth Time:

_____

_____

_____

Fifth Time:

_____

_____

_____

Intimacy Practice 8

Marie Kondo Your Love Life

THE QUICKIE BOX

HOW: Clean out your inner "closet," where you've stored your conscious and subconscious beliefs about love, sex, and relationships.

WHY: By letting go of the beliefs that don't serve you well, you are free to make your own informed decisions based on the values your adult self has adopted. This will give you the confidence to live your life in ways that are fully aligned with what feels right to *you*.

Our culture laughs at men who constantly want sex. We say, "Boys will be boys," or "It's just hormones," or "It's biological; that's how men are made." Too many people, including a lot of women, will ridicule anyone with a strong sexual desire. They act as if that desire precludes a sincere desire for a loving connection.

Honestly? I think that's bullsh*t.

I believe sexual intimacy is a powerful way to form a real, meaningful connection. Sadly, for many people, especially men, sexual intimacy is the only way they know to establish a personal connection. A great number of those people are also at a loss when it comes to using sexual engagement as a stepping stone to other intimacy, but I hope this book helps them figure out how to do so.

It would be foolish for us to overlook another category of widespread, sexually unhappy people: heterosexual married women. For many women, especially married moms, sex is a losing proposition—the chances of ultimate success are slim to none. Women who openly embrace their sexuality, relishing their body confidence and prioritizing sexy fun despite the demands of their kids or work, risk being ostracized by other women who deem them "slutty." Repressing their sexuality is likely to allow them to fit in with the other moms but doing so typically takes a toll on their marriage. In a very real way, women who fit in with "the women" find themselves being labeled "uptight" or "a bad wife" by their husbands. (How many women do you know who stay up to the wee hours of the morning, making cupcakes or decorations or _____, for a school event but refuse to consider sexy fun after 9:00 p.m.?)

Sadly, there are a zillion other ways that our actions and values can be at odds, but this exercise is designed to specifically address those pertaining to sexual intimacy. However, it can easily be adapted to address any other topics you'd like.

Have you heard of Marie Kondo? For a while there, everyone I knew was cleaning their house, thanks to Marie Kondo. She developed a method that encourages purging everything that doesn't bring you joy. To her, it's that simple.

Maybe it can be that simple for you too.

In her book *Spark Joy: An Illustrated Guide to the Japanese Art of Tidying*, she writes, "Life truly begins only after you have put your house in order."

While I hope she's wrong about putting your house in order—if not, my life still hasn't truly begun and probably never will—I do like to apply a similar approach to sexual intimacy.

If you're not wholeheartedly enjoying sexual intimacy or if you want more of it, taking stock of your thoughts, values, beliefs, and feelings about sex is a great place to start—especially since we are surrounded by very mixed messages that we internalize without noticing. We all have ideas from our parents, family, teachers, friends, and even the media that have probably infiltrated our consciousness at different times in our life. So it's no wonder we are often confused and conflicted about what's right for us.

The healthy thing to do is a deep clean! It's time to sort and organize the "closet" within you, where all of your beliefs about love, sex, and relationships live.

Right now, it might look like this (even if you're a neat freak, you've probably never noticed this hidden closet, so don't feel bad):

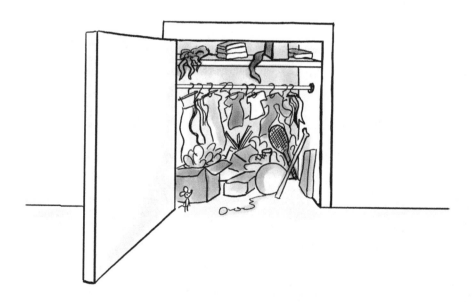

It's pretty easy to see the problem, right?

My closet has actually looked like that, so I speak from experience when I tell you that you'll feel much better by the end of this exercise!

In my very real, messy life, my favorite organizer insists that the first thing we do together is take every single thing out of the closet.

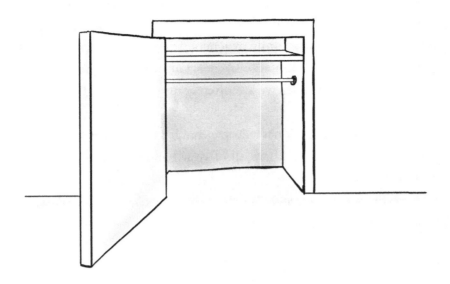

Then, and only then, does she begin the process of organizing. How? She lifts up every item, one by one, and we proceed through the following steps:

1. Does it fit me? Not *Did it fit yesterday?* or *Will it fit me tomorrow?* No, rather, *Does it work for me now?* Most of the time, my answer is, *I don't know! I have to try it on.* It's a slow, painful process for my ADHD self, but I know it's necessary if I don't want to live with chaos.

2. Once I try it on, there are a couple of options:
   a. If it doesn't fit, it doesn't go back into the closet.
   b. If it fits,
      i. and I like it, and it gives me joy, I find a place for it in the closet.
      ii. but I don't like it for any reason, it's not allowed back in!

This process guarantees that every day, when I'm deciding what to wear, my choices are items that fit and flatter me in ways that make *me* feel good. I no longer hold on to something just because my mother or boyfriend liked it or because someone gave it to me. My closet is reserved for my choices only. Of course, just because I like something today doesn't mean I'll always like it, so I always have the right to alter things or change my mind completely and get rid of it later.

Admittedly, this process is pretty much pure torture for me every single time (ADHD is real, folks!). But I know from experience that she is absolutely right: A clean closet makes every day easier because my options are clear. I don't have to second-guess everything I put on.

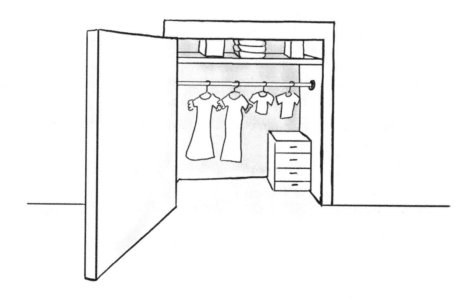

Now let's turn back to your hidden closet full of everything you've internalized about love, sex, and relationships.

Imagine yourself emptying it out completely, tossing everything into a nearby pile. Practically speaking, spend a week doing a brain dump by making a list of everything that comes to mind. Take time so that you'll have plenty of opportunity to notice your reaction to each thought. For example, you might be with someone who points out how much makeup another person is wearing, which reminds you that your mom once told you, "Only harlots wear bright-red lipstick during the day." Add that to your list *pronto!* (I've learned to love wearing bright-red lipstick at all times of day—sorry, Mom.) I find it helpful to keep an ongoing list handy because no matter how often I've done this exercise, I never run out of "stowaways," things that were so subtle it was easy to miss them until the bigger stuff was expelled.

Here are some examples of beliefs you might have in your closet:

- Marriage is a public sign that I am loveable.
- Sex before marriage is bad.
- Sex is dangerous.
- All men want is sex.
- Women make you "pay" for sex one way or another.
- Touching myself for pleasure is wrong.
- There's a right way for people to have sex and lots of wrong ways.
- It's wrong to have sex with "too many" people.
- My naked body is shameful.
- I don't like oral sex.
- Women aren't supposed to make weird noises or faces.
- I'm a pervert because I like _____.

Once you feel your closet is completely empty, you can actively decide what you *want* to fill your closet with, confidently discarding the rest. Here's an important thing to remember: just because you don't want it for yourself doesn't mean you're judging others who keep it.

When you start reviewing your list, it's usually easiest to begin with the big issues, regardless of the order listed. Start by choosing one specific thing at a time; then ask yourself questions such as these:

- What exactly is this? Is it a law, belief, value, rule, my grand-father's opinion?
- Where did it come from?
- Does it align with what I believe now?
- Do I believe that abiding by it will help me become the person I want to be?
- Is it something I want my children to learn?
- Does it help bring joy into my life?

It's best to do this sorting work alone so you can privately work through all the emotions it will bring up instead of being influenced by anyone else. After all, the whole point of this exercise is to stop giving free rent to others' opinions.

If there are matters you aren't certain about, keep track of them in another list that you'll tackle after you've finished everything else. It may be that the organizing process will give you the clarity you need to deal with these questionable issues. Or perhaps you will now have the confidence to discuss these issues with those you trust to shed insight, play devil's advocate, or otherwise support your efforts to uncover *your* truth—not simply give you their opinion.

Once you've dealt with everything you've accumulated so far, you can always add whatever new ideas, beliefs, or values you feel benefit you while having the confidence to dismiss whatever you think won't serve you well. You deserve to carefully screen everything, using your own belief system to ensure that your closet contains only what works for you, even if it's quite different from what you grew up with. Your belief system is entitled to mature, just like the rest of you.

Very few issues in life are as deeply personal or complicated as love, sex, and relationships, which is why it's not easy to erase a lifetime of lessons. Give yourself grace and time to organize yourself in this regard. Your life will be better for it.

Only when you are feeling confidently comfortable with your "closet" do I suggest you discuss things with your partner. Hopefully, they've been doing their own work at the same time, so you can have a shared "closet warming" party. The best part of this is that if you like what they have in their closet, you don't have to steal it; you can just magically duplicate it. Voilà! It's in your closet too!

On the other hand, you should expect differences; you're not clones! Discuss these differences with kindness and curiosity. Seek to understand why they believe such things as well as how they imagine these beliefs affect their life. Share your thoughts similarly with the intention of explaining rather than persuading. There's no need to reach an immediate consensus. Allow time for each of you to consider the other's perspective before revisiting the topics. If the differences relate to important aspects of your relationship and you're unable to resolve them on your own within a reasonable time frame, I encourage you to seek help from a professional coach or therapist. It's amazing how easy answers are to find for those not caught up in emotions.

What's really interesting about this exercise is that by choosing what we want to live with, we become more confidently capable of moving forward in ways that empower us rather than wear us down. My clients are often ecstatic about the changes they experience after they let go of the subconscious, limiting beliefs that have plagued them for years. They happily describe not only how their relationship improved but also how their life feels "easier" and "better" in ways they can't pinpoint but definitely notice.

For those of you who aren't in a committed relationship now, please don't wait to do this exercise. Not only will it help you be true to your own values while dating, but it'll also give you the insight needed to check out a prospective partner's "closet" before you become committed. This can save you a lot of heartache further down the line, so please make good use of it.

Lastly, here's a word to the wise: if your (prospective or current) partner isn't willing to do this exercise, it's likely that there's stuff hidden in their closet that they think you'll find stinky.

Again, it may sound weird coming from someone whose house is so cluttered—Marie Kondo would be scandalized! However, I know from personal and professional experience that while a cluttered kitchen can be ridiculously annoying, a messy internal love, sex, and relationship closet can be fatally destructive.

First Time:

_____

_____

_____

Second Time:

_____

_____

_____

Third Time:

_____

_____

_____

Fourth Time:

_____

_____

_____

Fifth Time:

_____

_____

_____

Intimacy Practice 9
Touch for Touch's Sake

THE QUICKIE BOX

HOW: Commit to 3 or more mutually pleasurable, consensual, nonsexual touches lasting 30 seconds or more, daily.

WHY: Intentional physical touch conveys affectionate connection and affirms trust while stimulating happy hormones that intensify positive feelings toward each other. It's like sprinkling pixie dust on your relationship.

Remember how, back in chapter 2, we talked about the science behind physical intimacy? Touch is remarkably powerful; it literally changes our bodies. Physical touch can amp up dopamine and serotonin (the "happy hormones"), create more oxytocin (the "love hormone"), and decrease cortisol (the "stress hormone"). Touch also decreases your heart rate and blood pressure. These are facts.

Touch for touch's sake (rather than as a means to initiate sexy fun) provides an affirmation of our connection that extends beyond the bedroom.

While there are lots of "easy" ways to touch, it's also easy to overlook the ways that touch becomes problematic for couples. Spooning together as you drift off to sleep together is one example that sounds sweet, but, much to my surprise, it is a source of conflict for many couples. The problem? The "big spoon" (the person cuddled around the other's back) often drapes their arm over their partner's tummy. That can feel really wonderful to both of you, unless the "little spoon" is sensitive about that part of their body.

Now, if that's problematic at the beginning of a relationship, it may not be hard for someone to say, "Hey, if you don't mind, I can't usually sleep this way." But if you've been doing it for the entire two years you've been together and it's only recently that your little spoon has developed a sensitivity about her midsection becoming a bit wobblier than she'd like, it wouldn't be surprising for her to be hesitant about speaking up. She probably loves the closeness spooning provides her, but that's now in conflict with her body image. She's tried to suck her tummy in, but that doesn't really work for long. Now she feels that being close to her partner is a reminder that she's not as "hot" as she was before. (Mind you, her thoughts may have nothing to do with what her partner sees, feels, or thinks, but they are important because they are her reality.)

This seems like such a minor issue, but what this couple does now will likely be part of a pattern that will last throughout their relationship.

With this in mind, let's get clear on the options available to this woman:

1. She puts up with it, trying to ignore her feelings so she doesn't flinch when he touches her stomach.
2. She explains her feelings to her partner, hoping he will understand them rather than dismissing them by telling her to just lose weight.
3. She can roll away when he spoons her, using excuses such as she's hot or the like.

How do you think each of these options is going to play out in the long term?

Just so that I'm being 100 percent clear, you are allowed to pick and choose what expressions of intimacy you enjoy. You don't have to do stuff you don't feel comfortable with as long as you find things that *do* work for you. Discomfort with one particular expression of physical intimacy is not problematic per se; discomfort with all forms of physical intimacy *is* a problem.

In other words, sucking it up and sucking it in are not likely to be effective solutions! It's healthy for you to be aware of any discomfort and to feel free to discuss it with your partner, even when it seems trivial. Mutual honesty allows for cooperative problem-solving, which fosters trust, comfort, and security.

Keep in mind that we all have vastly different backgrounds, baggage, and experiences. This affects how we interpret things. While some people think a slap on the ass is a love tap that conveys affection, others feel it's demeaning or an indication of sexual objectification. Personally, I don't believe there's an inherent right or wrong; it's context that informs my response. No matter where you find yourself in any given instance, it's important that you feel empowered to speak up in order to protect your boundaries.

Trigger warning: Physical intimacy can be difficult for people who have experienced trauma or abuse. In those cases, any kind of outreach, even the smallest touches, may cause a negative reaction. If that's you or your partner, I encourage you to move at a snail's pace, granting all of the power to approve or initiate touch with the partner who has previously had their boundaries violated. The goal is not to "tolerate" touch; it's to welcome or invite touch that empowers everyone while being confident enough to refuse those that don't benefit us. (If the idea of physical touch isn't appealing to you at this point, I suggest you skip ahead to the Just Say NO! exercise. This can be especially helpful for those of us who have previously been denied the right to say no.)

For anyone who is touch avoidant, scheduling even the smallest acts of physical intimacy with as much specificity as possible can provide a much-needed sense of control. "We're going to hug for two minutes while standing up in our living room every night at 9:00 p.m." "On Saturdays at 10:00 a.m., we're going to snuggle in bed for five minutes without any sexual activity (even if either of us becomes sexually aroused)."

Those examples may sound silly but knowing exactly what to expect in advance can make a huge impact by alleviating anxiety. It means that neither of you has to worry about being surprised, and it reinforces mutual trust. Because each of you is allowed to say what you want or don't want, it also prevents either of you from worrying about whether it's "good" for the other.

Deliberate, planned, and consensual touch can be extremely healing. Open communication and vulnerability about what feels good and what doesn't both serve to create a safe space where each of you can focus on relaxing into the pleasure of your tender, loving touches.

INSTRUCTIONS:

Deliberately touch your partner in an affectionate manner for at least a minute, three times a day without allowing your touches to be a precursor for sexual intimacy. You can either schedule your touches in advance or not, as you both prefer.

You may choose from the following options, but you're not limited to them, of course:

1. Hold hands while walking or watching TV.
2. Take a dance break together.
3. Pause for a hug when you pass each other in the house.

4. Brush your partner's hair.

5. Button your partner's shirt for them.

6. Take off your partner's shoes and/or socks.

7. Give a neck, shoulder, hand, foot, or back massage.

8. Kiss (mouth, neck, ear, hand . . .).

9. Tickle your partner.

10. Sit on your partner's lap.

11. Stroke your partner's face.

12. Walk or stand arm in arm.

13. Snuggle in bed together.

14. Kiss every time your team scores while watching a game.

15. Shower or bathe together.

16. Wash your partner's back or hair for them.

17. Dry your partner after a bath or shower.

18. Feed your partner with your hands, allowing them to lick your fingers.

First Time:

_____

_____

_____

Second Time:

_____

_____

_____

Third Time:

_____

_____

_____

Fourth Time:

_____

_____

_____

Fifth Time:

_____

_____

_____

Intimacy Practice 10

Can You Feel Me?

THE QUICKIE BOX

HOW: When you're not in the same physical place, verbally tell your partner *how* and *where* you would touch them, asking them to mirror that touch themself.

WHY: When physical intimacy with your partner just isn't possible, this is the best substitute I've found for physical touch.

There are going to be times when physical intimacy isn't possible for one reason or another. This can be problematic, especially when it's long-term. (COVID breakups were probably as common as COVID coupling!)

If you and your partner spend time physically separated, here's my advice: Acknowledge that physical distance takes a toll on your relationship. Even for those of you who don't typically engage in much intentional touching when you're together, the sight of your partner, or even their coffee cup by the sink, serves as a reminder to your head and heart of your connection to them. Their place in your life is affirmed. Subconsciously, you still feel attached.

"Out of sight, out of mind" sounds harsh, but there's a lot of truth to it.

The pandemic made it clear that video chats can help us feel connected despite the miles between us. But it also made it very clear that connecting virtually doesn't satisfy our need for the sensory, chemical benefits physical intimacy provides. While there are some clever sexual workarounds,[45] it's important not to overlook the need for nonsexual physical intimacy.

Just like we get hungry if we miss a meal, "skin hunger" occurs when we don't get as much physical intimacy as we're used to. Seriously. It's also known as *touch starvation* and *touch deprivation*.[46] Whatever it's called, it's real.

So what I suggest is that you conjure a little magic. Whether you're on the phone or on a video chat, you might say to your partner something like, "Hey, would you cup your face for me? That's what I would do if I were with you. I miss feeling your face. I want to feel your skin. When did you shave? This morning? Dang, I'd love to feel that stubble! Stroke your face for me, just like I would. Here, just do what I'm doing on my face so I can pretend it's actually yours."

The pleasure of this is twofold: As your partner strokes their own face, they get to experience how it would feel if you were the one doing it. Additionally, the physical sensations stimulate the hormonal benefits of your touch, even if they're not as intense. Directing self-touch is the closest we can get to physically touching one another when distance makes actual touch impossible. While it's not a perfect substitute, it provides huge benefits.

---

[45] I recently mailed a gift to a female friend before she went out of the country for a couple of weeks: an app-controlled vibrator that her partner could operate long-distance—even from overseas.

[46] Lauren Sharkey, "What Does It Mean to Be Touch Starved?" (Healthline Media, April 8, 2021), https://www.healthline.com/health/touch-starved.

There are some ways to take it even further.

Imagine saying to your partner, "I wish I could nibble on your ear. Can you put your fingers on your earlobe while pretending I am nibbling on it? Because that's what I want to do right now. Oh yeah! Now trace your lips with your finger as I'd do. How does that make you feel?"

Actually walk them through it. Where would you be touching them? How? With which body part? Your lips? Your fingers? Would your touch be soft or firm? Describe everything, every little nuance, down to the last detail.

This isn't the same as actual physical touch, of course, but it's a lot of fun! It's incredibly intimate, merging emotional and physical connection, which makes it deeply satisfying.

You can take this exercise in any direction you want. Make it your own special kind of fun. Get creative. Be sweet. Be silly. Be sexy if that feels right.

Here are a couple of examples of how my clients have created physical intimacy from far away:

William, who's been married thirty years, said to his wife, "The bed's empty without you. When I'm in the bed, I'm putting my hand out, caressing where your head would be on the pillow. Will you touch the back of your head for me? Caress it like I would, feeling how soft your hair is, savoring the warmth of your skin. Describe how you feel when I do it."

Georgina, who'd been dating her boyfriend for six months before he got sent overseas, told him, "If you were in bed with me right now, we'd be cuddled up, my butt squished into your crotch. Your face would be nuzzling my neck, your chin hairs tickling me. Can't you almost feel me doing it now? Am I getting a rise out of you?"

There's no wrong way to do it, although playing the song "Touch-A, Touch-A, Touch Me" makes it more fun for me! Go ahead, celebrate all the ways you'd be physically intimate with each other if you were in the same place. Let your imaginations run wild, fueling touchfests of epic proportions! Then, when you are in the same place again, do it all for real! Savor the gift of touch like never before.

Note: While this exercise can be as sexual as you'd like, I suggest you begin by focusing on the nonsexual intimacy. For lots of people, getting comfortable with long-distance touching can feel weird. These inhibitions tend to disappear quicker when they aren't exacerbated by any sexual inhibitions. (I can't count the number of couples who tried sexy Skyping, only to give up when one of them got cold feet a few minutes in.) When you're both completely comfortable with nonsexual virtual touch, adding a layer of sexy flirtation shouldn't feel as daunting. Building this up slowly is a way to avoid having someone shut down completely.

First Time:

_____

_____

_____

Second Time:

_____

_____

_____

Third Time:

_____

_____

_____

Fourth Time:

_____

_____

_____

Fifth Time:

_____

_____

_____

Intimacy Practice 11

To PDA or Not to PDA

THE QUICKIE BOX

HOW: Tell your partner what you are and aren't comfortable with. Be specific when explaining why you feel this way. Listen carefully as they do the same. Then find creative ways to satisfy the both of you.

WHY: How you appear in public as a couple impacts how others see you and can symbolize how each of you feels. This can be as important as how you're dressed.

I can't tell you how many couples struggle with the issue of public displays of affection, whether or not they discuss it. Interestingly, I don't see an obvious distinction along gender divides; in my experience, men and women are equally likely to crave PDA or hate it.

It's not usually the issue that brings people to me, but it's often the cause of underlying resentment, which means there's good reason for me to address it.

Obviously, PDA is a form of physical intimacy, but there's more to it.

It would be reasonable to expect that couples would figure out whether or not they share the same perspective on this topic during courtship, but no. It's much more common for us to get so caught up in the thrill of a new relationship that we overlook differences, minimize opinions that don't fit with ours, and tell ourselves that noted issues are minor, paling in comparison to the overall joy we savor.

Unfortunately, these minor issues are like a tiny pebble in our shoe that's easily ignored until the constant irritation has made us so sensitive that we simply can't stand it anymore. At that point, things are likely to get ugly as we explode, surprising our partner with our vehemence since they had no idea there was a problem.

My client Martine laughed humorlessly when I brought this up to her. She told me how a walk with her boyfriend on the Santa Monica Pier a year ago almost ended their relationship. She was feeling so loving toward him that she wanted to hold hands. But every time she took hold of his hand, he pulled away almost immediately. Her feelings were hurt and she couldn't stop thinking, *Wow, he doesn't even want to hold my hand. He must not want to be seen with me, or he must not find me attractive anymore. Either way, it really sucks.*

After all, she told herself, *he held my hand all the time when we first started dating.*

Instead of making herself vulnerable by sharing her fears and asking why he didn't want to hold her hand, Martine tried to play it cool, which, in this case, meant she said snarkily, "I thought we were going to have a romantic walk on the beach, but you won't even hold my hand anymore!"

This immediately put him on the defensive, so he snapped back something hurtful to mask his own wounded ego: "Well, I didn't want to hold hands then either, but you never gave me a choice."

Argh. I am literally shaking my head to get that image out; it's way too familiar to me, sadly.

For Martine, it was the start of a downward spiral that didn't end until we started working together.

In hindsight, that disagreement became the symbol of what was really wrong with their relationship.

It had nothing to do with handholding; it had to do with their habit of assuming what the other felt instead of asking.

If Martine had been able to ignore the voices in her own head long enough to ask her guy why he didn't want to hold her hand, he would have told her this:

"I used to hold your hand all the time because I was trying to show you how much I like you, and I knew it mattered to you. But after years together, I figured you know that I love you, so I don't think I have to prove it to you anymore. The truth is, I've never liked holding hands while walking because it makes my hand sweat, and it's annoying when there are lots of people to navigate around. I'm always proud to be seen with you; I just don't need to hold your hand to feel happy we're together. What I wanted, but felt silly suggesting, was to walk out to the water so we could kiss in the surf. That's what I thought would be hot." (In this example, hot and romantic are one and the same.)

To say that Martine was shocked by this confession would be an understatement.

Clearly, this isn't just about PDA; it's about how we choose to show up in the world as a couple. In turn, this has a big impact on how we feel in relationships. Whether we admit it or not, wanting to be with someone who publicly acknowledges their positive feelings about us and our relationship is almost primal.

Armed with this knowledge, you can recognize your desire to engage in or avoid PDA, asking yourself what doing so does for you: Does it affirm your connection, your commitment to each other? Does it feel constraining? Do you feel comforted or controlled? Get clarity so that instead of jumping to conclusions about your partner's take on things, you can use your words to describe what matters to you. Be brave enough to ask for what you want, offering options to make it easier to reach mutual satisfaction. There's no reason to treat PDA differently than your beverage preference at a restaurant. If it's included on the menu, you'll tell the server exactly what you want. If it's not or they're out of your first choice, you might ask for their recommendation after you describe what you want.

Telling your partner how you want to feel when you're together in public and letting them offer ways to make that happen makes both of you feel really important and truly loved. It can completely transform a frustrating stroll into a symbol of your commitment to each other.

PDA isn't just for new relationships.

First Time:

_____

_____

_____

Second Time:

_____

_____

_____

Third Time:

_____

_____

_____

Fourth Time:

_____

_____

_____

Fifth Time:

_____

_____

_____

Intimacy Practice 12

Pucker Up, People

THE QUICKIE BOX

HOW: Before you give a kiss, get clear about what message you want to convey. Ask yourself: What am I trying to tell them?

WHY: This helps turn your perfunctory pecks into purposeful pleasure! Remember: if you don't know what your kiss is saying, your partner won't either, so they won't know how to respond.

These days, kisses have been stripped of their power and potential. Too many people have exiled kisses into the realm of boredom. They've become superficial and meaningless. When I inquire about the frequency of kissing, clients tell me, "We kiss goodbye every morning before I leave for work," or "We always kiss good night!"

I get excited for them until I ask how they feel about these kisses. It's rare for me to get any answer other than something along the lines of, "Oh, it's just a quick peck, nothing to get excited about. But it's nice."

Cue eye roll.

Not really, of course. It's great to kiss your partner in the morning and/or at night! But generally, these kinds of kisses are perfunctory. A couple is just going through the motions. They're kissing superficially, out of habit, not with pleasurable intent. Sometimes it's a handy defense against unspoken concerns about their lack of connection: "Well, we still kiss every day!"

I don't mean to be dramatic, but I've yet to meet a struggling couple who kiss each other joyfully on a regular basis. The flip side of that, in my experience, is that couples who don't enjoy kissing aren't thoroughly enjoying their relationship either.

So if you're happy together, keep kissing! If you're not so happy together, start kissing!

REMEMBER: BE DELIBERATE WITH EVERY KISS!

Quick kisses are fine. They can be sweet and loving. But even those should be deliberate and focused. Each kiss, regardless of how long it is, should matter. It should register in both of your bodies and both of your hearts. Otherwise, what's the point?

Kisses should be more than just about touching your lips to someone else's. They deserve a "special sauce": feeling, intention, desire, affection, laughter, whatever you're feeling at the moment. Heck, maybe you kiss them in an unexpected place as an easy way to add some romantic intimacy.

One of my favorite quotes ever is from Mae West: "A man's kiss is his signature."

Isn't that brilliant? I'd only add that this is equally true for all of us, not just men.

That quote inspired me when I was dating a really cool guy named Noah. Problem was, Noah was a terrible kisser. Even though I liked him, I was on the verge of breaking up with him because I just couldn't stand kissing him![47]

---

[47] You know what's way worse? My "wasband" *never* liked to kiss. Not even during sexy fun! I should have run for the hills from the get-go, but I was so insecure I thought it was about me.

But before I did that, I thought, *What have I got to lose? Maybe I can teach him.*

I spent a week or two thinking about what makes a good kiss, and it finally hit me. So the next time I saw him, I asked him one simple question: "What are you trying to tell me with your kiss?"

Totally baffled, he just looked at me. He had no idea as to how to answer that question.

"I don't know," he finally replied.

"Well, then," I replied, "how am I supposed to know how to respond?"

That was it. That was the whole conversation. Noah got it. That's all it took. From then on, kissing him became a true pleasure, which, not surprisingly, led to other pleasures.

If you aren't sure what you're trying to say with your kisses, I'd suggest that getting clarity will improve your game dramatically. In fact, a fun way to test your skills is to play a guessing game with your partner.

"Okay," you tell them. "I'm gonna kiss you. Your job is to decipher what I'm saying."

Even if you already love the way your partner kisses, this is a fun game that will add a new level of meaning to your kisses.

As "Play It Again, Sam" sang in *Casablanca*, "A kiss is still a kiss." Just don't forget that every kiss can mean something different!

First Time:

_____

_____

_____

Second Time:

_____

_____

_____

Third Time:

_____

_____

_____

Fourth Time:

_____

_____

_____

Fifth Time:

_____

_____

_____

Intimacy Practice 13

The Love Seat
Home of the Cuddle Huddle

THE QUICKIE BOX

HOW: Carve out a safe, comfortable place where you and your partner can go to regroup, revitalize, and reconnect.

WHY: Every relationship deserves a "home base" that's protected from the struggles of the world, where intimacy is prioritized to reinforce your commitment to each other.

Just like athletic teams have locker rooms where the members can relax outside of the public's view, relationships deserve the same. That's why I recommend the following activity to everyone: create a love seat in your home.

If you're someone who is already chomping at the bit to go hit up your nearest antique store, feel free. But the rest of you can relax. This has nothing to do with buying a piece of furniture commonly known as a *loveseat*.

What I'm talking about is a "love seat" of your own making. It doesn't even have to be furniture. It can be anything—a cozy nook, a daybed, a balcony, the guest room's shower, the corner of a room. I've even had clients in small homes use a closet as their safe place.

All that matters is that you carve out a safe, comfortable place where you can ignore the world while focusing on yourself, your partner, and your relationship. It's a safe harbor necessitated by the fact that the "real world" tends to overlook the need for relationship maintenance, constantly demanding your attention to other (often less important) issues instead.

No matter how great your relationship is already, regular retreats to your love seat can make it better.

The point of creating a specific love seat is to designate a place within which you are the person your partner fell in love with, the one who also fell for them. When you enter the love seat, you leave your other roles outside. You're no longer the mom who organizes the family's to-do list or the dad who shepherds kids to baseball practice. You're not the one who's working a demanding, misery-inducing job. You are simply a lover seeking solace, connection, and joy by spending time with your beloved.

Your love seat can be your own romantic hideaway, providing sanctuary even in the midst of your hosting Thanksgiving at your house for twenty of your family members. No matter how insane things get, you can make a quick escape before blowing your top!

The rules for this space are very straightforward:

1. Within the love seat, the focus must remain on each of you as a romantic partner and/or on your relationship. "I hate that this dinner is going to drain me so much that I'm going to want to crawl into bed to cry instead of wanting to snuggle with you" is okay to say, but "I expect you to do the dishes after dinner because I'm going out for a drink" is not.

2. Any and all conversations must be personal in nature, not merely logistical. This means that "Please keep Aunt Bitsy away from

me before I lose my cool" is allowed, but not "How is Bobby going to get home from school tomorrow?"

The love seat is an escape from the world where you can be with, support, and love each other without getting caught up in the practicalities of life. Use the love seat as an emergency escape by whispering, "I need you at the love seat in two minutes," knowing that your partner will do everything in their power to be there. Then you can bitch, vent, commiserate, or simply hug each other tightly.

Wouldn't it be amazing to know that any time you want a "zap" of goodness from your partner, you can get it? Think about what having an exclusive shared space adds to your relationship. It's like a lover's version of a clubhouse! Members share the following: Trust. Connection. Vulnerability. Safety. Honesty. Closeness. Support. Escape. Fun. Commitment. Loyalty.

Regular visits should help energize you both to deal with the rest of life, knowing that your relationship just keeps getting better and stronger. When things are tough, the love seat will become the place you long for, providing a much-needed respite.

I frequently describe what happens in the love seat like a football huddle, but way better. Think of the love seat as home of the cuddle huddle! It's your relationship retreat, where cuddle huddles help you cool off, simmer down, or recover from a hard hit. You're reminded that *you* matter, not just as a parent, employee, sister, friend, or spouse but as a human with a loving heart. You can't help but be proud that you were chosen as a teammate by someone you love dearly. Cheering each other on is not only uplifting but also a privilege. The love seat can become the heart of your home.

Here's how to build your love seat:

1. Designate a specific location with your partner, preferably a space that isn't often used by others.

2. Use whatever you like to decorate your love seat with your partner, helping it reflect or honor your relationship. Cushions, pictures, blankets, and snacks are a few ideas.

3. Schedule regular meetings of at least ten minutes weekly. (Sunday mornings work for a lot of people, but choose whatever days and times are best for your schedules.)

4. Feel free to invite your partner to as many "surprise" visits as you want.

5. Always do your best to accommodate your partner's requests for visits to the love seat.

6. Respect the love seat rules in good times and bad. When you do, it will certainly help improve things.

First Time:

_____

_____

_____

Second Time:

_____

_____

_____

Third Time:

_____

_____

_____

Fourth Time:

_____

_____

_____

Fifth Time:

_____

_____

_____

Intimacy Practice 14

Back to Back, Skin to Skin
(a.k.a. B2B, S2S)

THE QUICKIE BOX

HOW: Take off your shirt and sit back to back, skin to skin with your partner. Each of you takes turns talking for 5+ minutes without a response from the other.

WHY: You'll feel liberated in saying what you need to say without holding back.

If you are someone who loves when restaurants suggest wine pairings, I'd like to invite you to enjoy this exercise in conjunction with The Love Seat: Home of the Cuddle Puddle exercise (Intimacy Practice 13). They go together like oysters and Chablis or, if you prefer, a tender cut of filet mignon with a velvety Bordeaux.

This exercise is as simple as it sounds: sit back to back, skin to skin while talking.

That's right. It's all about making the most of your conversations. It's not about aimless chitchat, though that might be what gets things going. It's the kind of talking that includes exposing our hearts, conversations that foster deep levels of connection.

It's funny how skin to skin takes talking to a whole new level.

There's a ton of research on the importance of skin-to-skin contact, all of it confirming that touch is powerfully beneficial at every age and stage of life. In the context of your romantic relationship, it's absolutely magical.

This exercise is super simple: Sit back to back with your partner, skin to skin. Then start talking.

Obviously, this means shirtless, preferably braless. (However, if being braless is so uncomfortable that it's distracting, keep it on.) The goal here is to maintain as much skin-to-skin contact as possible while you lean against each other, supported by the other. This is easiest when sitting on the ground, but if that isn't comfortable, you can try sitting on a small ottoman, straddling a bench, or whatever else you can think of.

From the moment you sit together, take notice of how the other responds. Tune in to the feel of their skin pressed against yours. Pay attention to whether you're relaxing or resisting leaning against each other. Focus on your pulse and breathing; is it in sync with that of your partner?

Check in with yourself. How do you feel about your partner's providing you with physical, tangible support? Does it feel good to know you're supporting them? Is it scary to think they're dependent on you?

Just because this exercise is simple doesn't mean it's not hugely impactful. My clients are often skeptical at first, but they quickly become fans. The reports I hear most frequently are along the lines of "It was so strange; I had tears running down my face" and "I felt closer to them than I had in years." One of my personal favorites is "It felt strange to be leaning on her."

I know you've probably been told time and time again that making eye contact is important during conversation because it lets people know that you're paying attention. This is very true. But there are lots of conversations that are easier, and more touching, when done *without* being able to see each other's face.

Back-to-back, skin-to-skin conversations allow us to say things that need to be said without worrying about our partner's reactions.

I'll never forget the moment, many years ago, when I asked my husband for a spanking. Before he uttered a word, I saw all sorts of emotions flash across his face. I interpreted them, rightly or wrongly, as fear, shock, and judgment. I wasn't thinking about the question from his perspective; I took it all on myself. I felt immediately ashamed because *he* seemed ashamed and embarrassed.

More than anything, I wished I'd never opened my mouth, so much so that I never asked for anything else in our marriage—despite our being married for twelve more years!

In a back-to-back, skin-to-skin conversation, having to talk nonstop without anyone watching our face generally causes us to let our guard down. We'll find ourselves saying things that take us by surprise and take our partner by surprise as well. Until you try it, you may not realize how much you're affected by facial cues from others.

Rightly or wrongly, we gauge interest, approval, and sympathy by what we see on someone's face. Consciously or not, we tend to censor ourselves when speaking face-to-face. We see the negative side of this freedom in the rise of cyberbullying. I much prefer to make use of the power in a positive manner. It's easier to say things like "I don't want to have sex because I'm afraid I can't stay hard" or "I'm afraid you hate my body since I gained/lost weight" without having to meet somebody's eyes.

For this practice, you'll have to set aside fifteen to thirty minutes.

INSTRUCTIONS:

1. Schedule at least one weekly B2B, S2S session to minimize the number of times either of you has to hear the dreaded "We need to talk."(But know that either of you can call for an urgent session whenever you want.)

2. Flip a coin to see who talks first or alternate each time.

3. You can agree on a theme for the session, like childhood experiences, an upcoming vacation, or whatever else is top of mind, or you can allow free flow. However, you must keep talking for your entire time allotment. Keep in mind that your focus should be on *your* feelings and reactions, not on logistical planning or giving the other person advice. (It's always interesting to hear what's revealed when people have to keep talking.) Note that there is to be no "rebuttal" to what the other person says until the final round.

4. Each of you takes a turn talking for the agreed-upon time—at least five minutes, but ten is better. Set a timer for each of you so no one has to watch the clock.

5. Once each of you has had your uninterrupted opportunity to talk, you can decide whether to allow an additional five or ten minutes to address what the other said or to allow back-and-forth conversation for the remaining time.

6. Feel free to ask for more time if you want but try not to be upset if your partner doesn't want to do this. (Refer to the Just Say NO! exercise—Intimacy Practice 6—if this is tough for you.)

Easy peasy, right? You can schedule the time so nothing else crowds it out, and then for fifteen minutes, you just talk. Talk uninterrupted, stream-of-consciousness style. You might start with mundane stuff, for example, "There's not much going on this week" or "The weather sure is hot!"

As you go on, you'll loosen up. You'll drop down into a more honest, vulnerable place. You might say, "You know what? Last week you did this thing, and I really liked it. So thank you."

Or maybe your partner will say, "You know yesterday when you left the house without kissing me? Maybe it didn't seem like a big deal to you but I thought about it all day."

Perhaps you'll say, "I hate my job. Every day I think about quitting but then I'm terrified you'll be upset."

A few years ago, I worked with Brandon, who used a back-to-back, skin-to-skin conversation with his husband, Nate, to confess something he had been keeping to himself for a while. He said, "I know we planned this trip to Yellowstone, and I'm excited about it. But the truth is that we've gone to a national park every year since we met. I'm dying to have an adventure with you in some romantic city we've never been to before. I should have told you before now, but I was afraid you'd think I was selfish since I know how much you love Yellowstone. I'm not trying to ruin our trip. I still want to go because I love traveling with you. But next year, can we change it up?"

When I saw Brandon afterward, he was practically giddy.

"I don't think I could have done it if we'd been face to face," he said. "I was too afraid he'd get that defensive look on his face that he always gets when he feels like I'm criticizing something he's done. I just knew he would say, 'I didn't make you say yes to Yellowstone! Why didn't you tell me? Why do you always wait until the last minute to tell me you don't want to do something?'"

Brandon laughed before adding, "Actually, he probably *did* have that look on his face. But I couldn't see it, so I just let it all out without stopping. Plus, it felt so good that he didn't argue at all. When it was his turn to talk, he just said he was glad to know how I felt and he'd be okay doing something different next year!"

You know what's cool about this exercise? The more often couples have B2B, S2S conversations, the more forthright they become in all their conversations. They get so used to being calm, cool, and supportive about even difficult things that it becomes natural, even face-to-face.

For Brandon and Nate, this step began a complete transformation in their marriage; neither had ever experienced such deeply rewarding emotional intimacy. Both vowed to never again settle for less. Oh, you'll also be pleased to know that the following year, they took a wildly romantic trip to Istanbul.

I never fail to be impressed by how the physical intimacy of one partner's skin against the other's as they support each other creates a foundation from which emotional intimacy can grow. That's why I think of the intimacies as an elaborate tango; it's a physical, emotional, sexual, romantic, and spiritual experience.

First Time:

_____

_____

_____

Second Time:

_____

_____

_____

Third Time:

_____

_____

_____

Fourth Time:

_____

_____

_____

Fifth Time:

_____

_____

_____

Intimacy Practice 15

Pleasure Pull
(A "Too Tired to Think" Game)

THE QUICKIE BOX

HOW: Each partner creates a container of sexy fun ideas they love, as well as contributing to a shared container of date night themes from which the couple pulls weekly to inspire their date nights.

WHY: This exercise will ensure that mutually satisfying sexy fun becomes a regular, easy, enjoyable part of your life, even during the busiest of times.

Being tired or not getting what you want aren't excuses anymore, thanks to this exercise. Instead of having to figure out how to please your partner, you just have to do what they've asked. Weekly date nights won't be the "same old, same old" anymore because you'll alternate responsibility for planning them based on ideas you've each contributed.

Supplies Needed: Paper, pens, and three small containers.

INSTRUCTIONS:

- Each person writes at least ten specific sexy things that they love on a piece of paper. Then they fold it, dropping it into a container labeled with their name. Here are some examples:
    - Giving or getting a back massage
    - Engaging in particular sexual positions
    - Holding hands on a walk
    - Giving or receiving oral sex
    - Taking a bath together
    - Showering with each other
    - Snuggling while watching a movie
    - Getting or giving a foot massage
    - Being kissed from head to toe
    - Orgasming and going right to sleep
    - Receiving or watching a lap dance or striptease
    - Participating in a passionate make-out session
    - Talking dirty
    - Being fed grapes and wine in bed
    - Sleeping naked together

- In the remaining container, they each contribute "themes" for sexy things they enjoy, such as the following:
    - Having "wham, bam, thank you ma'am"-style penetrative sex
    - Engaging in lights-on sexy fun
    - Having a candlelight picnic (indoors or outdoors)
    - Slow dancing together in the living room
    - Skinny dipping
    - Watching erotica together
    - Watching a romantic movie together
    - Getting dressed up and going out on the town

- o Having naked movie nights
- o Role-playing (such as doctor/patient, sexy cabana boy or housekeeper/hotel guest, plumber/broke client, etc.)

- Every Sunday:
    1. Each of you gives your partner a "pleasure pull," picking one random slip from their pleasure container. You must fulfill your partner's pleasure desire as detailed on the slip sometime during that week. Failure to do so requires that you do two pleasure pulls from the other's container the following week, which, along with the overdue pleasure, must be fulfilled in a timely manner.
    2. Additionally, one of you (alternating weekly) pulls a theme from the third jar, which becomes that week's date-night theme. The person who pulled the theme is responsible for planning the date night.

NOTES:

- If logistics make a particular pleasure pull or theme impossible that week—for example, you can't get a babysitter—then pull again until you draw one that is workable. Keep in mind that being tired or waiting until the last minute to try to find a babysitter is not an excuse!
- If you prefer to plan ahead, you can assign a particular day of the week for each person's pleasure and/or your date night.
- Bonus pulls are big wins for both of you. These can be granted by either of you as desired. You'll find that giving your partner an extra pleasure pull is a great way to make up for a lousy day at work.
- If you like friendly competition, you can create categories such as sexiest setting, most exciting or unique date night, or most

enthusiastic giver, awarding prizes to the winner at your own erotic award show!

- Caution: While it might be tempting to fill your container with sexy ideas that your partner isn't into for one reason or another, I suggest, instead, that you focus on activities comfortable for both of you. After all, this game is voluntary. You'll have a better chance of its continuation if you make it exciting but not over the top. You don't want to get into a "fooled me once but never again" situation. Plus, couples who make this game a regular part of their love life discover that their mutual trust grows with every pleasurable week they share. Before they know it, they find themselves naturally becoming more adventurous together.

First Time:

_____

_____

_____

Second Time:

_____

_____

_____

Third Time:

_____

_____

_____

Fourth Time:

_____

_____

_____

Fifth Time:

_____

_____

_____

Intimacy Practice 16

Fantasy Island

THE QUICKIE BOX

HOW: Let your imaginations run wild! Take turns sharing your turn-ons with your partner and then trying to make some part of the other's fantasies come true.

WHY: It takes a lot of vulnerability to share our turn-ons. Therefore, mutual sharing creates trust, and embracing our partner's desires creates shared pleasure.

Week 1: Each of you finds or makes up at least one fantasy video/ story that you find exciting and erotic. You can find inspiration by searching online for erotic stories, poems, and movies, or imagine an adults-only version of your favorite G-rated movie. Plan a date to share these with each other. When you've finished, tell the other why you chose that particular fantasy and which three parts of it you find the sexiest.

Week 2: The winner of a coin toss makes one or more of their partner's fantasies from Week 1 come true. This doesn't have to be literal, of course; if it's a pirate fantasy, maybe it's having sexy fun on a boat or while wearing an eye patch, etc. If it is a threesome, but you're monogamous, you could spend an evening talking about whom they'd choose for the third, as well as what they'd want to do with them. In short, take as much artistic, sexual license as you want! The idea isn't to be exact; it's to have fun and encourage creative sexy exploration together.

Week 3: It's the other person's turn to make things happen.

Week 4: Schedule a sexy, romantic date to discuss the activities. Talk about what was hot and what was not. Laugh together about how hard it is to be vulnerable enough to share the things that turn us on. Recognize that turn-ons don't abide by societal mores or political correctness, but that doesn't mean they can't be lots of naughty fun! Celebrate the fun you had by expressing your sincere thanks for trying something new—even if it wasn't a sexy success; share what made you giggle or feel nervous and appreciate that you feel safe enough with each other to try new things together, even if it's scary to do so. Talking about what happened, even the bloopers, will leave you with the memories of the fantasy fulfillments. You'll also have increased your level of emotional intimacy by sharing your feelings about what happened. Ding, ding, ding! Another big win for you both!

Bonus: Repeat as often as you want with new and/or updated fantasies!

Note: This is a great way to build anticipation for a truly romantic, sexy vacation or, after the fact, to keep your vacation memories alive!

First Time:

_____

_____

_____

Second Time:

_____

_____

_____

Third Time:

_____

_____

_____

Fourth Time:

_____

_____

_____

Fifth Time:

_____

_____

_____

Intimacy Practice 17

Lickable, Luscious Lust and Laughter

THE QUICKIE BOX

HOW: Make your own fantasy ice cream sundae!

WHY: Laughter is food for the soul—and potent medicine for a relationship.

I want to close with one of my favorite exercises. When we think of it as "sexy fun" rather than "sex," it's not goal-oriented. Fun is the only aim. That's it. Sexy fun has to be enjoyable. It should also be safe, joyful, and liberating for everyone involved.

What's one of the most frequently overlooked ingredients of sexy fun?

Laughter.

You already know I'm a big fan of laughter, but I'm not alone. Studies show that couples who laugh together stay together.[48]

---

[48] Laura E. Kurtz and Sara B. Algoe, "Putting Laughter in Context: Shared Laughter as Behavioral Indicator of Relationship Well-Being" (Wiley Online Library, August 24, 2015), https://onlinelibrary.wiley.com/doi/abs/10.1111/pere.12095.

Unfortunately, however, for many adults, laughter has become painful and more associated with being laughed at than the joy of laughing together.

Reclaiming laughter is one of the quickest and easiest ways for even an estranged couple to bond.

Taylor and Jordan learned this lesson reluctantly. By the time I met them, they'd been together for more than fifteen years. Like with so many of the couples I talk to, sex had become a painfully loaded topic. There was little of it and certainly no joy in it anymore, no lightness. Consequently, Taylor and Jordan felt frustratingly disconnected.

I was pleased with their forthrightness, their lack of defensiveness. They quickly acknowledged that the sexual intimacy in their marriage was lacking and had been for some time, but both accepted responsibility instead of passing blame. It's always a good sign when my clients are able to be vulnerable with me. It usually means they're willing to be vulnerable with each other too.

> Reclaiming laughter is one of the quickest and easiest ways for even an estranged couple to bond.

"You know what I want you two to do?" I asked, after they'd given me a pretty good sense of the current state of affairs.

They both leaned forward in their chairs.

"I want you to make ice cream sundaes."

Taylor was definitely the jokester of the relationship, always quipping and making witty observations. It was a delight to watch Taylor's face light up at this idea.

Jordan, on the other hand, gave me a look that could melt ice (not to mention ice cream!). Amusingly, he was a career foodie—as in a well-known food consultant and cookbook author—and definitely the more serious of the two.

"What kind of sundae?" he asked.

"I want you to get all the ingredients you'd use to make your favorite sundae of all time," I said. "Ice cream, of course, and then cherries, bananas, chocolate crumbles, whipped cream, syrup, even sprinkles. Go wild! Get whatever makes you drool with desire."

Taylor looked intrigued, but Jordan was skeptical.

"Can the ingredients be organically grown and locally sourced?" he asked, making me laugh.

"Absolutely, they can. This is *your* fantasy sundae. In fact, you're going to put them in the most organic place of all."

"Where's that?" Taylor asked, curious.

I grinned. "On each other."

It was Taylor's turn to burst into laughter. Jordan looked like he might have a heart attack.

"I'm serious," I said. "You're going to put down a sheet or a tarp or whatever you have on hand. Then you're going to use the other person's body as your "bowl," where you'll create your fantasy sundae. Make a mess. Take pictures if you want. Rub each other all over. Use a spoon or lick it off. Anything goes. Most importantly, laugh a lot. Have tons of fun. I'm serious, but this exercise isn't! Get over yourselves and be silly for a change. Have some good old-fashioned fun together for the first time in forever!"

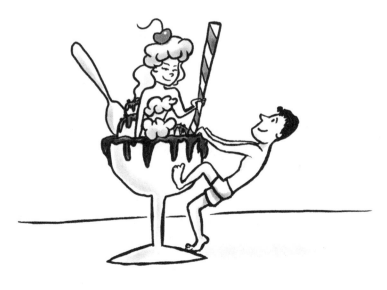

When they left their session, I could see that Taylor was grinning, but Jordan was less than thrilled with me. I figured there was only about a 50 percent chance they'd follow my advice, so I was surprised when, just a few days later, Jordan called me.

"I really thought you were nuts," he said. "But Taylor convinced me to give it a try. I was right; it was crazy, but we laughed more than we have in *years*. Beth, I have to tell you: Taylor was the best sundae of my life."

I smiled for the rest of the day. Frankly, I smile every time I think of them. I never get tired of love and laughter.

First Time:

_____

_____

_____

Second Time:

_____

_____

_____

Third Time:

_____

_____

_____

Fourth Time:

_____

_____

_____

Fifth Time:

_____

_____

_____

CONCLUSION

Happy Endings for All

I love a good happy ending, don't you? It's what I want for all of us.

But over and over, I see how easy it is for couples to sabotage their own happy endings, even when they love each other dearly. Even when all they want is to be happy together forever.

> The secret is to get closer. In hard times, create *more* intimacy instead of less.

It hurts my heart when disagreements, tension, and struggles arise—as they do in life—and one partner starts pulling away as if that can protect them. Sadly, the typical response is for the other partner to respond in kind, which reinforces the perception that the relationship isn't a safe place. So, one painful step at a time, each withdraws from the other. They increase the distance, often retreating into themselves to lick their wounds or, worse, to mount a strong defense.

The worst part about this is that the solution is absurdly simple.

The secret is to get closer. In hard times, create *more* intimacy instead of less.

As long as you eat right, sleep well, exercise regularly, and have lots of intimacy, you should live a happy, healthy life!

Remember that the 5 Kinds of Intimacy are vital to keeping your love alive.

Here's a quote I love from Dr. John Gottman: "In any interaction, there is a possibility of connecting with your partner or turning away from your partner. One such moment is not important, but if you're always choosing to turn away, then trust erodes in a relationship—very gradually, very slowly."[49]

Take this to heart, please. If you're usually good at physical intimacy, add more. If your partner is depleted and not meeting your desire for sexual intimacy, give them whatever kind of intimacy they crave most until they are "fully charged" again. Generally, partners want to be good to each other, so why not make it as easy as possible for yours? If you give what you can as often as you can, your love has the best chance of thriving.

The exercises I've shared here, when used regularly, can be reparative or preventative. There's never a bad time to employ them. When you commit to maintaining healthy levels of each kind of intimacy at all times, you should have enough goodwill to sustain your relationship, even through difficult times.

Have a cuddle huddle for just a few minutes every day to reconnect.

Carve out a little time for reverse spooning so you can reclaim a shared perspective.

When being vulnerable with each other feels impossible, take a leap and go back to back, skin to skin for a conversation that might be difficult to have face to face.

I can't wait for you to experience the fantastic transformation that so many other couples are enjoying because of this revolutionary new approach to intimacy. I encourage you to try all the exercises, even if you think they're weird. I promise, they've all been used by a wide

---

[49] Nadine Clay, "Turning Toward Your Partner Instead of Away Will Improve Your Relationship," Medium (P.S. I Love You, August 3, 2020), https://psiloveyou.xyz/turning-toward-your-partner-instead-of-away-will-improve-your-relationship-1bdadceb0035.

variety of couples, all of whom have found that they added more love, joy, laughter, vulnerability, closeness, and—of course—intimacy to their relationships. I know they can help you to enjoy the passionate, loving relationship you've always dreamed of.

But wait! If what you've read in this book is meaningful to you, there's no need to say goodbye!

I couldn't fit everything into this book (according to my editor, anyway), but I've got more for you if you're interested! I'm offering *free* exclusive content to all readers, including additional exercises and work-sheets to help you continue to explore, expand, and experience more of the 5 Kinds of Intimacy. To get your *free* bonus worksheets, use this link: BethDarling.com.

Also, I'd love to connect with you online so we can continue the conversation. I invite you to friend or follow me on Facebook, Instagram, TikTok, and YouTube. Plus, if you like fun, naughty conversations about the bare-naked truth about love, sex, and relationships, I invite you to subscribe to my podcast, "Come With Us Podcast." For those of you who want to become more comfortable with your sensual, sexy self, I encourage you to read my book *Love and Laughter: Sexy (Meaningful) Fun for Everyone.*

I hope you're feeling a sense of accomplishment and pride for having taken this deep dive into intimacy with me. In fact, I want to give you a kick-ass compliment!

You are *amazing*. Seriously. You are someone who takes your love and life seriously. You're willing to open your mind to new ideas, learn new tricks, and perse-vere—even in the face of more than two hundred pages! Truly, you are my kind of people, and I'm thrilled that you took this journey with me. Please wrap your arms around yourself and give

> It's the beginning of a love that stays alive and makes your dreams come true.

yourself a big squeeze from me 'cause that's what I would do if you were here.

You deserve so much more than a happy ending. You deserve a romantic relationship that is healthy, deep, real, vibrant, passionate, meaningful, sexy, and fun.

Because, in truth, this isn't an ending.

It's the beginning of a love that stays alive and makes your dreams come true.

With an abundance of love, hugs, and gratitude,
Beth ❤

P.S. If you liked this book, I'd be hugely grateful if you'd take a moment to leave a review on Amazon and/or Goodreads. Every review reminds the algorithms to suggest this book to others who are searching for relationship advice. Thanks for helping me share happy endings to all!

P.P.S. I've got so much else to share with you! :-) Keep reading for details.

Want More Beth?

Get a **FREE** Bonus Intimacy Practice to make sure you never run out of ways to keep your love alive by joining my mailing list at BethDarling.com

Tune in to my weekly podcast: *Come With Us Podcast* (available wherever you get your podcasts)

Read my other book: *Love and Laughter: Sexy (Meaningful) Fun for Everyone*

Connect with me directly on social media:
- Facebook: https://www.facebook.com/bethdarlingsexygenius
- Instagram: https://www.instagram.com/bethdarlingsexygenius
- TikTok: @bethdarlingsexygenius
- YouTube: https://www.youtube.com/c/DarlingWay/videos

Email me about speaking engagements, workshops or 1:1 coaching services: Beth@DarlingWay.com

ACKNOWLEDGMENTS

I've wanted to write books about love since I was a kid, but I had no idea it was such exquisite torture. Not just for me as the author but for all my friends and family. I'm beyond grateful that they have loved and supported me throughout this long, stressful, sometimes incredibly difficult journey despite the fact that I dropped so very many other balls along the way. I owe y'all more than just this shout-out, but at least I'll start here. 😊

While I am convinced that preaching and teaching love, sex, and relationships is my calling in life, I can't ignore the fact that this is sometimes "awkward" for my kids. They know so much more about their mom's personal life than most people are comfortable with, but the upside is, from my perspective, my relationship with each of them is more intimate and fulfilling than I ever imagined possible. I'm forever thankful for all the thoughtful feedback they gave me at every stage of this book, from challenging my theories to editing drafts, even helping me choose the cover. Kit, Kelsey, Quinn, Kaliela, and Kiya, thank you for being such amazing people with huge hearts. You are the biggest blessings and best parts of my life; I love you with every fiber of my being.

One of the most unexpected pleasures of this book was sharing parts of the draft with my "wise beyond her years" teenage granddaughter; her feedback not only warmed my heart but was truly insightful. While my grandson is far too young to read anything yet, his huge, bright smiles when he saw me on video calls energized me on even the most frustrating days. I now understand the power of a muse! Aeri and Kirby, being your Bubbe is a joyful privilege beyond measure.

Of course, there's no way you'd be reading this without the patient brilliance, skill, and devotion of my developmental editors, Bree and Christopher, and Redwood Publishing's Sara Stratton. I'm grateful for not only their magnificent writing skills but also their ability to wrangle my ADHD, stream-of-consciousness writing style into a fun, easy-to-read book. It's more than accurate to say that working with them forced me to refine, sharpen, and clarify my theories overall, making them more impactful for readers and clients alike.

As a reader, I had no idea how many people with different skills have to pitch in to create a good book, but believe me, I do now! I'm fortunate that Avery went above and beyond as copyeditor extraordinaire to make sure that readers could enjoy a smooth read on their journey through the book. I'm indebted to Kelley Sweet (Photography) for carving out time for me in the midst of her busiest season and then refusing to settle for the "easy shots"! It's thanks to her that those of you who "picked up" this book because of its eye-catching cover photo are here. (And I'm so glad you are!) Michelle Manley of Graphique Designs then worked her magic, turning a stunning photo into a compelling book cover. Not to be outdone, Toonimal's illustrations are a much-appreciated visual delight. Lastly, Redwood Publishing as interior designer is the one who put all these parts together in such a way as to create a book not only worthy of your time and attention but also your pleasure. There are no words to convey my gratitude to each of you.

I am forever grateful to my remarkable friends Gary Krupkin, Tia Kansara, Joe Marich, Jody Monkovic, and Julie Torrant for not only reading early drafts of this manuscript but for respecting me enough to give me the seriously valuable, constructive feedback I needed. It's thanks to each of you that this manuscript got exponentially better so quickly. I adored each of you before this, but this level of trust is uniquely special and beautiful. (But don't worry, I take full responsibility for any new or remaining issues!)

Also, to my dad, siblings, and other family members who have been on the receiving end of my pursuit of more intimate relationships, whether they liked it or not. (Special thanks to Uncle Sandy, who said I was the first woman he'd ever talked to about sex in ninety-five years, and he enjoyed it!)

Lastly, I can't begin to recognize all the clients who have trusted me to be part of their love stories, as well as the legions of other friends and family who have encouraged me to persevere even in the midst of my own doubts, fears, and failings. There's not a doubt in my mind that without your affirmations and confidence, I would never have had the guts to write this book. I owe you everything, but all I can give is my heart.

XOXO,
Beth